T0149328

GETTING BETTER

Healing Prescriptions for Patients,
Families and Friends

Mark Landiak

authorHOUSE®

AuthorHouse™
1663 Liberty Drive
Bloomington, IN 47403
www.authorhouse.com
Phone: 1 (800) 839-8640

Published by AuthorHouse 04/04/2016

ISBN: 978-1-5049-8421-8 (sc)
ISBN: 978-1-5049-8420-1 (e)

Library of Congress Control Number: 2016903855

Print information available on the last page.

ACKNOWLEDGMENTS

Thanks to all who provided inspiration and content for the writing of this book:

My writing advisor, Dan Campana, who listened to me ramble on for hours on end and managed to help me get my words down on paper.

Megan, Dara, Denise, Lucie, Amy, Denise, Sarah, Kelly, Kyra, and all the nurses at Edwards Hospital along with: Lesi, Rose, Brian, Nikki, Laura, the other Laura and the entire team at Loyola Medical Center. You are truly the best. And, the caring team in the Edward Cardiac Rehab Center as well.

The team of physicians who have given me, and those who continue to give me the best of care and caring: Doctors: Bakhos, Baughman, Costanzo, Franklin, Greenstein, Nemivant, Pappas, and Sweiss. I'd really appreciate it if you all can figure out how to keep me around for a long time to come.

All the people who advised me and helped to keep my business healthy when I wasn't: Dino, Bill H, Bill C, JB, Chad, Cody and especially Meg who has been holding it all together for 25+ years.

My best friends who keep me laughing throughout the toughest of times and are helping me get through all this with a smile on my face: Dave ("Pimpster"), "Murph," "Ringo," George, Eddy J., "Sick Jim" and Joe Z.

All my soccer friends who have encouraged me along the way, especially: Gary, Ted, Tony, Ed, Paul, Jim, Kevin, Rick, Mike and Mike and all the guys in the Half Century Club. I hope to be with back to my old form on the pitch one day!

My Faith team: Father Pat and Deacon Joe and the countless people who've sent prayers my way. Keep 'em coming.

My amazing, 95 year-old mom and dad who I get to see almost every day and continue to be amazed with for their vigor, smarts and love for one another after 70 years of marriage.

My awesome sisters who were always there when I needed them – even though they live 700 miles away.

My incredible family – Nicholas, Elise, Olivia, Luke, and my wife Barbara - You all are truly the lights of my life. I love you all more than you'll ever know. And especially to Barbara…I'll bet you never imagined that "through sickness and in health" meant you'd have to endure the "sickness" part to this degree.

This book is dedicated to all those suffering from the a
effects of serious injury or illnesses, and
To my father, Nicholas Landiak,
a member of the 8" Scar Club and one of the
most resilient human beings I've ever met.

Sarcoidosis is a rare disease thought to originate in the immune system, which can attack multiple organs in the body. The effects are horrible and it is a disease for which there currently is no cure. Research funding is minimal because of the rarity of the illness. Please consider making a donation to this organization. 100% of all donations and a large portion of the proceeds from the sale of this book will go to the Foundation for Sarcoidosis Research. You can make a donation by going to the FSR website at: StopSarcoidosis.org

To leave a comment or order additional copies of *Getting Better*, visit: GettingBetterWithMark.com

A friend shared with me that the word "healthy" consists of the words Heal and Thy...as in:

Heal Thy Heart
Heal Thy Body
Heal Thy Mind, and
Heal Thy Soul.

Guess there's plenty of healing to go around.

INTRODUCTION

I never expected to get seriously ill.

If you are a fellow patient, I'll bet you didn't either. You ask yourself, "What do I do now?" If you're a family member or friend, you were likely surprised to hear that someone you care about is really sick and are probably wondering what you can do for the person faced with serious illness.

Once everyone involved is over the initial shock (which can take some time), you look for ways to make it better and cope with the situation. Lots of questions run through your head. For example: "How do I remain in a positive state of mind despite the circumstances?"

When you or someone you know falls ill, you learn how the power of a well-placed "I love you" or even the exchange of a hug, or a glance and a smile can make a difference. Maybe it's just a call to check in or an email that picks up the spirits. You also learn about your faith and how to strengthen it if you choose to do so.

Whether you are the patient, the family member of someone who is very sick, the friend of someone going through an ordeal with their health, or a caregiver, you can make a difference.

You learn a lot about life when you are faced with the possibility of an early departure. Early departures are great if you are one of those folks who is perpetually late for everything (and you know who you are), but not so good if you are a patient.

When you become "a patient," life as you knew it changes and takes on a whole new look. You learn how to take care of yourself differently, so you can function as best you can despite the circumstances. Unfortunately, many of us learn all this the hard way.

A few years back, I contracted a rare disease called Cardiac Sarcoidosis. It came on suddenly and hit me like a ton of bricks. It is particularly aggressive and unfortunately, there is currently no cure and very little money for research. At this point, the best a sarc patient can hope for is to keep it at bay and that is what I work on every day. Very few people have ever heard of Sarcoidosis and I've learned that it is rare enough that many doctors don't know much about it either. It is an auto-immune disease that prevents the body from reducing internal inflammation causing scaring in vital organs and often resulting in organ failure. Sarcoidosis most often attacks the lungs and my doctors don't know why it showed up in me and decided to attack my heart. A large percent of the time, it moves to infect multiple organs. I'm fortunate to have a great team of caregivers working on my recovery. I'll tell you about them in these pages. My pledge is to live my life as best I can, and try to smile my way through the mental and physical challenges of being sick and working through the healing process. Making the best of your situation or helping others to make the best of their situation is what this book is all about.

To the last point, while in the hospital and recovering at home, I did many things to keep my sense of humor as a means to cope with all that was happening and the gravity of the situation for my family and myself. I'm not promoting my approach as something you should do, just sharing what is working for me as I'm trying to deal as best I can, with a very serious illness that may never go away. I started journaling many of my thoughts and the things I saw and did that made me smile, or even laugh out loud. I brought this philosophy with me into the hospital and when they sent me home. I've had over 100 tests and doctors "visits" since this all began. It can wear you down if you let it. I've learned a lot about the healing process through the experiences of others and through my own unique ways of staying happy despite the circumstances.

Those situations helped to form the basis for this book. I boiled the process of getting better down to five categories that we all can have some control over: Faith, Family, Friends, Fitness & Fun. Those elements became the foundation for how I now live my life and for this book. I also came to learn that anyone can harness any or all, of these five elements to feel better. Getting Better isn't meant to be a cure or substitute for medical care – it is a collection of stories and ideas that make the healing process easier and more pleasant for all involved. And some of it might actually make you "feel" better.

Once at home, I learned how challenging it can be to fight off the frustrations of being ill and how you really have to work at remaining positive and staying focused on getting better - not to mention communicating to the people who care about you, how they can help you through this process.

Getting Better is as much for family and friends as it is for patients. My hope is that other caregivers (doctors and nurses) will find it equally entertaining and enlightening as they look at the impact they can have on the quality of life for those they care for … and care about.

So this is my story. It covers my experiences during the first 5 years of my illness. My hope is that something in these pages will bring you some comfort and maybe encourage you to employ a few of the ideas into your own plan for helping yourself or others with Getting Better. One more thing. During the writing of this book, my father got very ill and he too now faces a life-threatening situation. This taught me that it is very different to look at the healing process from the foot of someone else's bed and I will try to be sensitive to that as well.

And, while the topic is serious, many of the stories in this book are intended to bring a smile to your face. So, feel free to smile and even laugh out loud if you like, as laughter is indeed a strong medicine. Okay then, if you're ready, let's get better.

THE ASCENT

In March 2011, I woke up at the bottom of the Grand Canyon, one of my favorite places on Earth, in a tent next to my oldest daughter, Elise. It was our third day of backpacking, and little did I know it would very nearly be my last.

The Grand Canyon is an amazing place with its breathtaking, panoramic views and sheer expanse. If you don't believe in God when you arrive, you might just be converted after a day or two of witnessing His majesty spread out before you as far as the eye can see. In fact, one can hear people professing their faith all over the canyon: "Oh my God."

As beautiful as it is, hiking the Canyon can be rigorous and dangerous. For this reason, most people don't hike to the bottom or on the lesser-known trails. We did.

As a father, I couldn't ask for much more. My daughter chose to spend her final college spring break backpacking in the Grand Canyon with her dad instead of whooping it up on some Florida beach with her friends. I've done one-on-one trips with all four of my kids, but hiking the Canyon was an activity reserved for Elise and me. We'd done it a couple times before and were both in good enough shape to do an even longer exploration this time around...or so I thought.

I was still floored to think she wanted to be in this wondrous place with me. Every day, I think I am the luckiest dad in the world and now more than ever, I'm reminded how much I love my kids every time I am with them. On this occasion, there we were, crammed into a small tent at the bottom of the Canyon, with the sound of Clear Creek and the Colorado River bubbling in the background. It was our final night and I thought about what a great time we had together. In the morning, we'd planned to hike out of the canyon and back to everyday life.

We woke up early, excited for the challenge of powering up the steep South Kaibab Trail that would take us to the canyon's rim. I wasn't at all prepared for what was about to happen next. Just as we started up the very first steep climb of the 8.5 mile trek out, something began going terribly wrong. My legs fatigued. My breaths shortened. I began to perspire profusely. My heart raced. We were less than 20 minutes into a hike of what should have been about 4.5 hours and my body was already wasted.

I rested a moment and drank a bottle of water disbelieving I could be in serious trouble and thinking that I was dehydrated from the 14 mile trek on the previous day. I seemed to recover and started off once more. 15 minutes later and BAM! It hit me again. What was going on? I'd never felt like this before. Imagine having the worst case of the flu you've ever had and attempting to climb the 2,109 stairs of the Willis (Sears) Tower in 85 degree heat…then having to do it 10 more times.

As I continued to struggle, Elise became more and more worried. She walked behind me, often with two hands on my pack pushing me up some of the steepest trails in the canyon, carrying her pack and supporting mine. She offered to take my 60-pound pack, but I wouldn't let her. At 22, Elise had grown from daddy's little girl into a physically fit young woman who was an accomplished soccer player and was training to run her next marathon. If ever I appreciated her athleticism, it was in this moment. Elise, on the other hand, probably wished at that moment she had decided to hang out on a beach watching the spectacle that has become spring break instead of witnessing the spectacle of her dad's situation. She was more than worried and thoughts were running through her mind that dad might not make it out.

We saw no one for the first two hours of the arduous ascent out of the canyon. We were alone and I was in big trouble with no phone or cell phone service to call for help.

As I was relaying this story to Dan Campana who helped me get all this down on paper, he wanted to talk to family and friends about their view of each situation. You'll see a number of their comments scattered throughout the book. Here is a comment from my daughter:

"There were some times when I was really scared. We're in the middle of nowhere. I've never seen him like that before. It wasn't until he started wobbling and not talking that I thought we might have to get help. I was making emergency plans up in my head."-Elise telling Dan about the experience

I kept looking for milestones – make it to that corner, get to that rock, keep moving toward that tree – Elise looked at my colorless face and had to wonder whether I was going to leave the Earth right then and there. And, I might have if not for her presence of mind and strength to push me up the steepest climbs. She may well have saved my life that day.

Upon reaching each of these small goals, I'd rest on a rock, take a drink and recover enough to begin the push to the next milestone only 200-300 feet away. This went on until we finally emerged over 8 hours later. Setting goals and beating them are part of life for many people. It's a mindset used to win in sports, build successful businesses or just to be the best

3

possible person you can be. It's the approach I've used for athletics and work. It helped me get out of the canyon alive and I've used milestones every day since to help heal my mind and body. I've learned that no matter how dire your circumstances, there is always a milestone you can reach that will put you a few steps closer to getting better.

Oddly, within 2 hours of finishing the hike, my body recuperated as if nothing had happened. I attributed the whole episode to a severe case of dehydration, something all too common that gets plenty of people into trouble in the Canyon. I was in denial, and why not? I'd always been in great health. Up to that point, I'd never been sick aside from the occasional cold. I'd always been in great shape. I was invincible. Or so I thought.

Little did I know that a very dangerous disease had just sent me a pretty obvious warning that it lurked inside my body and was ready to let loose. Like many testosterone-filled, ego-oriented males, I ignored the incident. What an idiot! I had just dodged the first of many bullets.

> *"There was no mention of going to a doctor. Just*
> *a lot of 'glad-we-made-it-out' jokes."- Elise to Dan*
> *about the post-hike conversation with her dad.*

THE DECLINE

Three weeks later, "recovered," and undeterred by the Canyon experience, Genius Boy (that's me) tried to run a 5K race with my two sons. About 400 yards into the race, something didn't feel right and I had to slow down to a jog, then a walk, then stop. Undaunted, I gathered myself, then pushed on with the same result. I even tried to gut it out by power walking to build up to a run. The same thing happened again and again. Every time that I started running, I'd immediately lose energy – I crashed about 20 times during that race, but did I stop? No. Duh. What was I thinking? After all, I'd never been sick before. (Oh, wait...Hey Mark, remember the Canyon three weeks earlier?) Let's do the math: one near death experience plus another near death experience equals go see a doctor. I should have called an ambulance. I felt horrible and knew something was very, very wrong. (Another bullet dodged). The next day I still felt awful and that was enough to put me in a doctor's office that afternoon. When my doc saw the EKG, I was in the hospital the next day. Now for the first time in my life, I was officially a patient.

Surviving the canyon and the ill-fated race attempt marked the start of a much longer, more difficult climb out of the unfamiliar territory that I found myself in. Over the next 10 months I underwent nearly three dozen hospital and lab tests. They did almost every heart and lung test known to medicine. Nothing. They then looked at my liver, kidneys and gall bladder. Again, nothing. While doctors and specialists poked, prodded and groped my fifty-something year old body, I continued to get worse....a lot worse. So bad, in fact, that I could not make it up one flight of stairs without stopping and looking for a place to immediately sit down.

Let me put that into some context: I've always worked out to keep myself in good shape. Played soccer twice a week, went on many long runs, never smoked, and drank in moderation (except for some "best forgotten" incidents in college). Now, things got so bad that even attempting a slow walk down the driveway to get the morning paper left me completely exhausted, out of breath and unable to keep going.

After the internist, the cardiologist, the pulmonologist and various other specialists, the neurologist was next. She diagnosed me with Myasthenia Gravis, a neuromuscular disease which originates in the auto-immune system. She referred me to a second neurologist, a supposed "specialist" from Northwestern University, one with more experience with that disease. He offered his own (incorrect) diagnosis. He said I had Lambert Eaton Myasthenic Syndrome. That's what he treated me for over the next six months, ignoring the negative test results, the worsening symptoms I was having and not caring enough to check with some of his associates about my case - despite my request for him to do so. And all the while the real disease was destroying me from the inside. (That was a huge learning experience. If you're not getting better and your doctor isn't talking to other doctors about your symptoms, fire him or her and find another doctor. That's what I should have done about 6 months earlier. This guy was all ego and no action).

By Fall, 2011, the high dosages of steroids and inactivity were helping me to feel a little better. My youngest son, Luke, played high school water polo, so I'd take him to the health club where he'd swim to get in shape for the upcoming season. There was a racquetball court there, so while he was swimming, I killed the time by hitting the racquetball around by myself. It had been many years since I stepped on the court in my past life as a tournament-level player, but I enjoyed the practice and my skills came back quickly. So I decided – like a fool – to enter a tournament. I hadn't played a competitive match in over 5 years. Something is drastically wrong going on inside me. I know there is a big problem…and something inside my head tells me to enter a tournament? What was I thinking?

Since I'd been feeling decent enough to practice, I thought that maybe I could exercise my way out of my illness. Yeah, that was another classic brainstorm of mine. So I thought getting into this competition could be good and I wanted to relive my glory days. Since the neurologist from Northwestern who was supposed to be taking care of me was no help whatsoever, I was building my own Monthly Treatment Plan. What I forgot – beside, you know, almost dying and being unable to walk up a flight of stairs just a couple months earlier – was how intense and vigorous competition can be. I had no business being out there. Still, I'm a hard-headed Ukrainian. As my sister says, "You can always tell a Ukrainian … you just can't tell him much."

So, I'm in this tournament and by the end of game one, I knew something was definitely wrong. Again, I thought I could work through it. Michael McDonald wrote a song about this. *"What a Fool Believes."* It was my theme song back then. So, after a long hard fought point, I get hit with a tsunami. Can't breathe… In a cold sweat… My heart is pounding on the inside of my chest like a misbehaving child who wants to get out of his room. I looked up at the ref, but could not speak. My face was void of color and I was blacking out.

One look at my face and the ref knew something wasn't right. He immediately called 911 for paramedics. I staggered out of the court, barely, and collapsed two steps outside the door. I had never felt worse in my life. The only thoughts in my head as I lay on the carpet were of disbelief – I can't believe this is happening to me – that and, I need to fight to stay conscious. The Grand Canyon didn't kill me, and I sure didn't want to die outside a racquetball court in Lombard, Illinois.

Every fiber of my being wanted to pass out, but no way was I going to let this happen. I fought as hard as I could. Somehow I knew that if I blacked out, I wouldn't wake up. I couldn't speak and was barely coherent. I felt someone pounding on my chest administering CPR. I couldn't move and did every relaxation technique I could think of to settle my racing heart and, the next thing I know, I'm staring up at five paramedics. It must have been a slow afternoon, because the entire Lombard Fire Department showed up. I'm sure glad each and every one of them did.

They quickly hooked me up to an EKG. One of the paramedics reading my EKG said it was the worst that he'd ever seen. They couldn't believe the readings, so they repeated the test. I laid on the floor for 45 minutes and consumed about a gallon of water while they continued to monitor my vitals. Defibrillator paddles were at the ready. They didn't want to move me and I didn't want to move. Slowly, my body started to recover. I had very nearly died, but said no to an immediate ambulance ride to the hospital. Despite strong urgings to the contrary, I signed a form validating my decision to decline the hospital trip as I wanted to get to my own hospital and my own doctors. I think the back of the form required another signature to validate that I was an idiot for not going right then and there, but I don't remember exactly. Another 90 minutes or so passed, and I recovered enough to get up and walk around – just like my rebound after the Canyon ascent, but a lot groggier. I stuck around another hour, ate a slice of pizza (the universal recovery drug) and drove myself home. But something was different this time. I was really sick. I don't know how I made it home because I don't remember driving home. I passed out (literally) in my bed and slept for 12 hours straight.

A wake-up call came first thing the next morning from my cardiologist, who had the results of a heart monitor test from the day before my racquetball court collapse. He ordered that someone drive me to the hospital immediately. Yes, I did have a heart monitor test on the day before the tournament started…but, I didn't have the results yet, so I made the decision that it would be OK to play. In my defense, I actually believed that this might be good for me. My Cardiologist, Dr. Pappas, said I was having 50,000-70,000 extra heartbeats per day and probably had been for several months - plenty enough to kill anyone. But, this time, being a stubborn Uke and in good physical condition worked in my favor. I can't help but believe that God had His hand in this as well. He probably called St. Peter over and said, "hey, check this one out. I've been sending this guy blatant signals for almost a year and he still doesn't get it. Should we bring him in?" Then St. Peter probably said something like: "That's amusing. Let's keep him around a little longer just to see what ridiculous thing he'll do next?"

After an MRI at the hospital, a team of doctors conferred and concluded that I had something called cardiac sarcoidosis, a rare heart condition where inflammation in the heart creates scar tissue that, in my case, affected the heart's electrical system and created wildly erratic contractions (ventricle tachycardia) which prevented it from pumping blood properly. The disease is particularly aggressive and gets progressively worse. Tests showed the right side of my heart was severely enlarged from the strain I was putting on it. They immediately implanted a pacemaker/defibrillator in my chest to keep me alive. Cardiac sarcoidosis starts in the immune system, but where it comes from is a mystery. I don't fit any of the profiles for someone who typically gets it. That didn't matter. With my new diagnosis, off to intensive care I went. The next thing I know, I'm waking up with a highly sophisticated device in my chest, and wires running throughout my heart.

This crash course learning experience taught me three really important things:

1. If your body is sending you some pretty obvious signals, and especially after your next near death experience, for goodness sakes, go immediately to the Emergency Room.

2. If you doctor isn't helping you get better (like Dr. Ego, my ex-neurologist), there are plenty of competent ones out there who actually care. Find them. And,

3. Regardless of how bleak your situation might be, hang in there because God might just keep you around, if for no other reason than you are a source of amazement. The real learning is that He likely has a bigger plan for you, no matter how many signals you miss. (Can't you just see God and St. Peter up there shaking their heads and saying. "He entered a racquetball tournament? Really?!")

MIDNIGHT INTRUDERS

So there I was, laying in the Intensive Care Unit of Edward Hospital staring up at the ceiling thinking: What am I doing here? I've been battling this unknown disease for almost a year and now I was truly fighting for my life. Like many patients, I wasn't at all prepared for the experience and was still in a state of denial.

Hospitals, especially the ICU floors, can be very scary places. They are not at all conducive to healing, which is ironic because that's what you supposedly are there to do. The healing process can become even more challenging when all you want to do is leave, but know that you can't. Fear and uncertainty can pervade. And what's worse is that people keep telling you to get your rest, but aside from the sleep clinics, which I'll tell you about later, hospitals are the worst place in the world to rest. It's nearly impossible to sleep through the night...in part because of the vampires.

The most intimidating people in the hospitals are not administrators, surgeons or, gasp, the collections department. They are the phlebotomists – a name that even sounds intimidating. Phlebotomist. It's a job title very few people outside the hospital or medical community have ever heard of, disguised to make you think they are something they are not, like "politician."

They can appear anytime, but usually sneak into your room when you are just about to, or have just fallen asleep. They will also come in to wake you any time that you have finally achieved deep slumber, often at 4 or 5am. They are relentless and undeterred from their mission to stab you with their needles and extract your blood.

These descendants of Dracula appear innocuous enough when they tap lightly at your door. Such a pleasant knock that you might think it's a loved one stopping by to visit. By the time you say, "Come in," it's too late. There they are. You see the cart carrying your floor mate's blood, along with brightly packaged needles that remind you of the kiddie toys your childhood dentist would give you after a cavity-free checkup. But this is no kiddie toy. It's a package containing an instrument of bruising and pain – and it's sharp. At the times when they can't find your veins for some reason, it's more like a bayonet.

In all my years, I never met anyone who openly admitted, "I'm a phlebotomist." In real life, I think they remain incognito by choosing to tell people things like: "I'm in the import/export business" or "I work for a research lab."

I decided to make the best of my situation and keep my wits about me. One strategy to disarm the phlebotomist is with simple words. One of the vampiresses who entered my room and woke me at 4:45 one morning was surprised by my greeting: "Good morning, Kelley. Thanks for coming in this morning. How are you doing today?" Then I started in with some pre-dawn chit chat. I was about to beg for a reprieve, but sensing I had let my defenses down, she plunged her needle into my arm like a professional seamstress threading her way through the first stitch of a heavy wool garment. "Ouuchhh!"

After her job was completed, I hit her with: "Great job this morning. You're awesome." She looked stunned by my comment. "No one has ever called me that," she said flatly. "People hate me. I have the worst job in the hospital." I started to feel sorry for her, realizing she was right. In a moment, she finished, packed up the blood, apologized and went on her way. It must be hard having to say you're sorry all day for doing your job. Then, as she turned to close the door, I swear there was a little glimmer in her eye and the faintest hint of a smile on her lips. Of course, it had to have been because of my sparkling personality and quick wit so early in the morning ... or was it because she had successfully bitten yet another victim?

The early morning phlebotomists – Sharon and Kelley – were awesome for two reasons: They always kept their sense of humor, but more importantly, they always hit my vein on the first try. That wasn't the norm for several of the external lab people or anesthesiologist intern who felt taking blood or inserting an IV was an inexact science where two or three or five, yes five attempts was an acceptable success rate. Unlike in horseshoes and hand grenades, close certainly doesn't count when it comes to jabbing needles into someone. Just ask any patient with bruises up and down their arms.

CHANGING THE GAME

This rare medical problem of mine was my initiation into the bad health fraternity. Maybe you're a member as well. Well you're not alone. I'd never spent a night in a hospital before this disease entered my life. Hospitals can be intimidating and even a little scary. So, I had to reset the environment (and my head) to make it work for me, my recovery, and those around me. I knew that I had to focus on minimizing worry and stress for me and my family. And, I had to focus on getting better. That's why being friendly and joking around with the nurses became an important part of my daily routine. You see the nurses more than your doctors, so you might as well get to know a little about them.

Just about every time a nurse, doctor or blood sucker walks into your room they ask two questions: What's your name? What's your birthday? You'd think they could remember this after coming into your room 60 times each day. It didn't take long for me to catch on to that. At first, I'd tell them, "June 20th," then ask: "what are you getting me?" One day, a new nurse came in, but I beat her to the punch. "Hi, what's your name? ...What's your birthday?" I asked. We had a good laugh and it turned out her birthday was a few days away. So I asked her a few questions about what big plans she had and we joked about some of the things she might do. Interactions like this add a personal element into an otherwise impersonal environment. It can change the relationship to be more human.

Another endless ritual – especially for heart patients – is the check your vitals ritual. In the ICU, this occurs every one or two hours whether you need it or not, and despite being hooked up to more monitors than are in the control room of a nuclear power facility. A nurse's aide came in to check my vitals and I posed a simple question:

Me: Can you check my blood pressure on my foot today?

Nurse: No.

Me: C'mon, let's try it.

Nurse: No, it doesn't work.

Me: How about the calf, then?

Nurse: No.

Me: OK, try my thigh, and don't get fresh.

Nurse: You are an aggravator. Now, give me your arm.

Me: And, you lack creativity, but I still love you.

In the process of keeping things light – and we'll get deeper into it later – you give people a chance to lighten the mood of their job. Essentially, you are promoting them from employee to Caregiver. Some might roll their eyes, but when you rewrite the rules of a mundane "chore," it can become more fun and interesting for both of you. This also distracts from the pain, discomfort and stress of the situation. And even if they call you an aggravator, they might just look forward to the next interaction precisely because it won't be mundane. Whether you are a patient, nurse or any caregiver, you have a lot more control over how people are going to respond to you based on how you respond to them. Think of how much impact you can have on that person. I came to realize that maybe "getting better" wasn't just for me to work on as a patient, but also for me to work on with those around me who were trying to help me recover. And, if they take a little more interest as a result, it can make a big difference.

Consider the phlebotomist, I got her laughing one morning to the point of crying – although maybe she was in tears for another reason. Here's the thing, I don't want someone who's going to stick me with a needle at four in the morning to think she's got the worst job in the world and that everyone hates her. That could result in torture…for the patient. When you change the quality of the interaction from mundane to more enjoyable, you change their mindset. In the hospital, it's so important with nurses, because they come to see you so often. The nurses (and phlebotomists) at Edward Hospital in Naperville, Ill., are wonderful. Anyone who can cover 7 or 8 miles on the same floor over a 12-hour shift and still come into my room and say good bye or good night with a smile on her face is worthy of flowers in my book. Or since this actually is my book, worthy of a shout-out and a public "thank-you." They executed their jobs with a high degree of professionalism, gave me confidence with their competence, and, they humored me as I tried to entertain and heal myself during my initial 220 hour stay and subsequent sleepovers. Lucie, Megan, Dara, and Amy put up with me and helped me through a very difficult time. I get to see them on occasion during my volunteer work at the hospital and they always ask how I'm doing? and how's my family?

I also had a really good experience during my stay at Loyola Medical Center in Maywood, IL as well. Tish, Rose, Brian and Nikki took really good care of me. There was one nurse in the ICU who didn't seem to want to be there and it showed. Her inattentiveness and attitude made me feel downright unsafe. I had just emerged from open-heart surgery and was in a lot of pain. On top of that, the immediate hours after surgery is also a precarious time that requires full attention. Her attitude and lack of urgency made me feel worse, not better. I had to call her manager and request a change. Perhaps they moved her to accounting. What a difference it can make, especially when it comes down to having confidence as a patient, that the person in charge of your well-being is actually competent and that they actually care. It's a tough job and I have a new appreciation and respect for people when they tell me, "I'm a nurse."

SEND IN THE REPLACEMENTS

Now, I have a great team of doctors, but I noticed something when one of my regular docs would be off during the weekends and a substitute would stop by my hospital room. These replacement docs likely gave my charts a superficial glance before walking in. Fine. I don't expect them to take over my case. It's what they would ask – as innocent as it sounds – that got me snickering a bit.

"How are you doing?" the substitute doc or nurse practitioner would ask.

I always found it to be a puzzling question. Many times I thought of offering a sarcastic response along the lines of: "Well, I'm on the ICU floor fighting for my life and no one can tell me about my prognosis, but my heart-healthy breakfast was tasty, so overall, I can't complain. And, how are you doing?"

Here's the thing – Most of the time I didn't know how I was doing. To this day, I still don't know exactly how I'm doing. That's why I'm in the hospital or why I'm coming to the doctor's office: to find out how I am doing. Maybe tell me something like: "it's good to see you," and ask me how I'm handling the boatload of medications I'm on, or if there have been any noticeable changes since we last talked. Maybe it's just me, but I'm of the opinion that after hooking me up to every manner of medical technology, taking my vitals 12 times a day and constantly siphoning the blood out of my body for lab work,

SOMEONE should know how the heck I'm doing and give <u>me</u> that information.

I learned not to expect much from a courtesy visit by the subs. Beyond the inane question, stethoscope here and there, flashlight in my eyes, ask about pain, and we're done, you won't be any better or worse off. It finally dawned on me that they couldn't tell me anything because they didn't know anything about my history, complications, prognosis, treatment plan, etc. Every so often, one would channel a little Patch Adams and make me smile or laugh. I don't expect them to do much to heal me in that short encounter, but most did nothing to elevate my mood or reassure me in any way. However, I noticed later they did charge for their "visit." I wish I could go see people in my neighborhood and charge them for my visit. "Hi, I'm here on behalf of your next door neighbor friend who is away this weekend. <u>How are you doing?</u> OK, good. Well, it was nice visiting with you. Here's an invoice and I'll see you tomorrow."

THAT BED IS YOUR ENEMY

One of my early hospital tours lasted nine days, and, fill-in doctors aside, I was focused strongly on getting better from day 1. And, let me say that I am lucky to have some very good doctors on my team. My electro-physiologist is Dr. Eugene Greenstein. He was part of the team that saved my life and performed the installation of the souvenir pacemaker/defibrillator now embedded in my chest. Shortly after I awoke from the procedure, he came to me and said, "You need to get up. That bed is your enemy. I want you up and moving around as much as you can. Start by getting out of that bed and into that chair."

It was really important for me to hear that right then and there as I lay wondering what just happened and what would happen next. He lit the fuse on my healing process and from that moment I began asking about all the things I could do to get better...with doctors approval this time.

I've learned that we all have to find the things that give us strength and motivate us to reach our next milestone in the quest to get better. That "next milestone" mindset helped me get out of the Canyon and since then, helped me cope with the mental, physical and emotional canyons that come with being really sick. It can work for you, too. Even if you are confined to a bed, there are things you can do to elevate your mood and occupy your thoughts. Maybe you have an interest and decide to become an expert on something. Maybe you'll start researching your illness and treatment plans. Maybe you have a trapeze attached to your bed to help you up (or to do pull ups). Maybe you get on the phone and start reconnecting with old friends. Maybe you write a book. The point is to do "something" that will make you feel productive, happier, more accomplished or just better in some way. And if you are the friend or family member, just remember that you are part of the healing process for the patient as well. Patients are looking for: lots of prayers, a listening ear, a hand to hold, a positive comment, interesting stories, good jokes, warm hugs, and anything that will keep them comfortable and smiling instead of thinking about their circumstances. I'm fortunate to have several people to help me in that regard.

It's easy for some patients to be consumed by their situation. That can drain your emotional and physical energy and you need plenty of both to heal. If that's you, don't be afraid to let people know how you feel and try putting a few of the ideas in this book to work for you.

It's all very easy to say you're going to attack the problem and fight to get better. Frankly, when you first hear the bad news of what's wrong, it's enough to disable even the strongest person's resolve. That's what happened to me.

YOU HAVE GOT TO BE KIDDING ME

I used to love watching John McEnroe play tennis. He did it with a skill and intensity that was, at times, very over the top. Whenever a close call went against him, he'd storm over to the umpire and blast him – infamously shouting, **"You have GOT to be kidding me" or "You CANNOT be serious."** McEnroe would throw tantrums and racquets in some of the best sports rants of all time. (Check out McEnroe's tantrums on YouTube) Yet, somehow, he'd regain his composure and get right back in to the match. He'd channel his frustration into a ball of energy focused on winning. McEnroe was not going to let a call that he thought was bad keep him from yelling a bit or winning - and he won a lot. He'd complain a bit and then get back to business. I love the guy. Maybe, he'll read this and give me a call. When you're really sick, you get a lot of bad news. It comes with the territory. It's inevitable that we'll get calls against us. I think it's normal to react emotionally. Some cry, some get mad, some get depressed and some break their racquets (or something else). Do what you need to do. Vent if you need to. Then get down to the business of healing. Try to "win" every day by improving in some category…any category. At one point, I took just surviving the day as my win. I even told myself that getting bad test results were a win. "Well, it could always be worse. I could be…"

For 6 months, my neurologists were pretty well convinced I had a neuromuscular disease, but nothing they tried worked. All the tests they did came back negative or inconclusive.

What I learned from that is that if you aren't getting a straight answer from one doctor, ask another – perhaps in a different discipline. Not being properly diagnosed very nearly cost me my life. After my first stint in the ICU, I wasn't sure what was going to happen next. But, I was sure that I wasn't going down without a fight. At first, there were signs of improvement. Then the bad news kept coming. Then, some improvement, then a big backslide. One saying that I remember a business associate telling me years ago is: "Expect the best, but prepare for the worst." The ups and downs of the healing process wear on your resolve. As patients, we need to stay positive, and prepare our minds and bodies to do battle, to beat the odds, to win our health back or at least to have the best quality of life we can have given the circumstances. This is no easy task especially if you've been fighting the good fight for years and don't seem to be winning. When things were at their most critical, I was talking with my financial advisor and friend, Bill Hammond about the prospect of dying. I was preparing for the worst. Without missing a beat he replied: "We all could die tomorrow. No one has a guarantee on life. You're here today, so what are you going to do?" Wow. That brought things back into perspective very quickly. After all, I am still here. So, what can I do to make the most of however much time I have left? For all I know, I could make it into my 90's like my dad.

My circumstances are far from great. That said, they could be much worse. So, the question remains: What am I going to do to get better in some facet of my life? When the bad news was coming in weekly helpings, it always made me think about whether I'd ever be able to return to my job, play soccer, go for a run with my kids or take a long walk in the forest preserve with my wife. Receiving bad news can be traumatic and the first reaction is typically along the lines of *"You've got to be kidding me"* or that other McEnroe classic, "You CANNOT be *serious!"*

I felt that way while staring up at the ceiling and five paramedics outside that racquetball court. Prior to entering that tournament, I erroneously thought I was getting better. The new diagnosis was even worse than the misdiagnosis. "You've got to be kidding me." Then, six months after I left the hospital, just when I thought I might be getting better, the disease resurfaced with a vengeance. Here we go again. "You cannot be serious!"

THE MOST IMPORTANT QUESTION
TO ASK YOUR DOCTOR

Many patients reading this book have likely received unfavorable news at some point. We all react differently, but we all have one thing in common – none of us are happy about it. After we absorb the diagnosis (or lack thereof), it's easy to get depressed. Maybe we just hope that things will get better or even think about giving up. A more difficult, but more productive course of action is to channel your thoughts and energy toward finding ways to take an active role in your healing process to the point of doing something you used to be able to do and loved doing. This means finding something that will motivate you to push forward. It might only take a simple question to your doctor to develop your path and goals. *"Is there a chance that someday I'll be well enough to …?"* This can be the point where you find your direction. What are the things that you want to do most? All you need is to know there is a chance and keep working your way down the list of things you want to do until you get a "yes." For me, the question I kept asking was: *"Is there a chance I'll be well enough to play soccer again?"* At first, they didn't offer much hope. They didn't want to get my hopes up because my heart was such a mess. Heck, I couldn't even walk up 7 stairs at one point. They gave me a five year recovery window "if all goes well." That's what I needed to hear. A little over 4 years after the Canyon incident, I was able to return to the soccer pitch. My stamina is lacking and I move a lot slower, but I've never enjoyed the game more. The score doesn't matter to me anymore. My "win" is just being out there with my friends kicking the ball around. I now enjoy and appreciate every moment more than ever. And, there are few things more gratifying than achieving a goal that once seemed remote. At several points, the chances for recovery seemed remote, but success, at least at some level, was possible, so there was still something to shoot for. For my next milestone, I asked my docs if there was a chance that I could hike in the Grand Canyon again and they said it would be difficult, but possible perhaps a few more years down the road. So, I plan to return there some day and conquer the trail that conquered me. Often our milestones take much more time than we'd like. But, after all, that's why they call you "patient."

HELP YOUR DOCS

During the early stages of my illness, my two cardiologists and head cheerleaders were Dr. Maria Rosa Costanzo and Dr. Evans Pappas. They work for different groups, but communicated with each other about my case and gave me (and continue to give me) the best of care. Just as importantly, they gave me confidence to face my situation head on. They tell it like it is, but also tell it like it could be. It's so important to know the possibilities and whether there is the potential for a path back to health even if the road is long and difficult. And, I know they care about me and are doing everything they can to guide me through this. I think I drive them crazy with my journals, health updates and list of questions every time we meet, but I need to be prepared to get the answers I need and the answers I want to hear. I feel fortunate to have them working on my case.

I also learned that some doctors know how to fix things, but not the things that may be wrong with you. That almost killed me too. Helping to coordinate medical care is another thing that family members can help with – especially when the patient isn't in any condition to do it themselves. Bottom line is that you have to work hard at getting the information you need to get better. SO, the key is to get the information you need one way or the other and get second and third opinions when you're not seeing progress. You also need to get the doctors to talk to one another. It took me a year and a near death experience to get the right team in place. Now I have utmost trust in the doctors responsible for my care…and there are a lot of them. Some, like the pulmonologist, electrophysiologist, gastroenterologist and the internal medicine man, I now only see 1 or 2 times per year. However, I copy them in on my health report, so they are informed. Sometimes, they even call me right after they get it to toss in their two cents. After my collapse outside the racquetball court, I had 2 primary cardiologists and a rheumatologist coordinating my care and referring me to other specialists as needed. I was referred to a dermatologist as sarcoidosis can also show up on your skin and I was concerned about what looked like a small cyst on my eyelid. He took a biopsy of a lump on my eyelid and it came back positive. He referred me to a Mohs surgeon who had to remove half of my lower eyelid. He then referred me to another who did the plastic surgery to minimize the facial damage. The 3 of them talked, sent pictures, discussed my case and expedited the process, so I would not be in bandages at my daughter's wedding. Find the right doctors and they'll treat you right. By the way, I owe a shout out to Dr. Amjad Ahmad, the plastic surgeon who did an amazing job on my eye. He expedited things and went above and beyond for me. And, his staff were attentive, friendly and genuinely happy for me. Bottom line is that he did an amazing job and he and I had a great rapport despite the fact that he went to the University of Michigan and I went to Penn State.

THE BEST CASE SCENARIO

As a patient, you need to give your doctors the best data you can about changes in your condition, and always ask them about the best case scenario and what it will take to get there. Pay attention to your symptoms and log them. I've decided to take on the role of Physician's Assistant. Of course, I don't get paid and I only have a general idea of what I'm talking about, but I know what I feel and see, and report it all. Family members can help with this as they see changes in your condition that you might not recognize. I give a copy of my journal to my team of doctors every few months and before every checkup. At one point, I was sending 8 copies out. I've seen one of my docs only once, but he is brilliant and I send him updates as well. I figure that he might read something that triggers a new treatment strategy and give one of my other docs a call. My journal consists of the following:

- All notable Changes in my condition since last report. (1-2 paragraphs)

- Medication List (and any changes since last month)

- Status report for list of Ongoing and New Symptoms (Better? Worse? Same?)

- Exercise Regiment and effects (Could I do more/less than the last time we met?)

- Copy of recent tests and Lab Reports

- Changes in weight, blood pressure, overall well being

- Recent / Upcoming Appointments and procedures

- List of questions (this one is very important)

I send them my journal in advance and review it with them on every appointment. It makes for a much more productive appointment...for both of us. In one appointment, I noticed that Dr. Nadera Sweiss, my rheumatologist, had taken a highlighter and went through my report highlighting the things she wanted to ask me about.

If your doctors can give you a path to walking in the park again or simply being able to attend the next family wedding, then build your treatment plan around that milestone. If the potential is there, then latch onto it like a Rottweiler on a steak bone and work toward that end. Easy? No way. In fact, in many cases, the odds might be against you to make the kind of recovery you ideally want. That's my situation now. Still, I'm prayerful and determined to make the best recovery possible, so I work at it every day. There are days when you don't feel like feeling positive. You may be pissed off at your situation and start to wonder "why me?" I've found that these are the days when you need to get your game face on and decide to beat the odds. Try as you might, you can't do it alone. As strong-willed and ego-centric as I've been in my life, I realized pretty quickly after collapsing that getting better was going to take much more than I could do alone – it's not just up to me this time.

That realization, developed while sitting in my hospital bed, was accompanied by the idea of how I would need more than doctors and medications to cope with this ordeal and get better. I couldn't do surgery or prescribe medicine, so I had to find the things that I had some control over to help me get better.

THE F WORDS

Very simply, there's no way to know how quickly or how well your body can or will recover from what ails you. Some of us might never return to the same physical condition we once knew. Those with terminal illnesses face an entirely different struggle to find some type of wellness and the strength to face each day with dignity, grace and good humor.

What everyone can do is wake up in the morning and define success for that day. What can I accomplish? How can I win the day? Or at the very least – What can I accomplish/do today that will give me some sense of satisfaction?

During my misdiagnosis phase, I always wanted to push the envelope physically, but didn't know how far I could go. At that time, my case had been turned over to the neurologists who weren't much help in building a treatment plan. So with my vast medical knowledge and experience, I designed my own plan that had me slowly building myself up again: jog 100 yards, walk up 15 stairs, or even do 5 minutes on a piece of exercise equipment – none of which I could do at the time. I'd show the neurologist my plan for each week and he allowed me to proceed without monitoring the impact. Too busy to care I guess. That ultimately turned out to be a bad thing because of the additional damage I was unknowingly doing to my heart. Early on, none of the doctors knew what was wrong and I felt the need to do "something" because I wasn't getting any better. So, the lesson learned is to find good doctors, get second opinions and keep them informed. Ultimately, that's what I did. But, it took a near death experience to find them.

Since I had never been sick before, I cast my signals off as "something else." After all, "I don't get sick." Now I've moved 180 degrees in the opposite direction. I want to know what's going on. I want to know what the medical terms mean and I read the research. I get on the internet and talk to other patients with similar problems to learn what's working/not working for them. I want to know about the drugs I'm taking and their side effects. I want to know as much as I can to have a meaningful conversation with my doctor instead of sitting there pretending like I know what they are talking about. This comes naturally for me now, as I want to know everything I can and Google makes it pretty easy. You might be in a position where one of your family members or friends can help you in this capacity. Most of my doctors tell me that I'm more in touch with what's going on with my body than most patients. That's because I now see the responsibility for my health and well-being is as much in my own hands as it is my doctors. The big exception is the surgical part. I have no ambition to operate on myself, but do want to make sure the person who does has some level of competence and experience. I'm sure the first solo operation for some fresh, new 20-something year old with MD embroidered on his smock is a very exciting day for him or her, but for me…not so much. Give me the seasoned veteran who's done it 500 times. Some nervous kid with a scalpel is not what I'm looking for.

As the months passed, I just wasn't getting any better and came to realize (or admit) the severity of my heart trouble. I knew my future physical activity would be severely restricted. No soccer. No tennis. No running. Hell, I had to build up to a short walk up the block that wouldn't leave me too tired to get home with the dog. I had to reset my goals. In the hospital, initial success was getting my feet on the floor to get in a chair, then walking to the door, then down the hall, then walking the entire floor, then doing it twice.

Doing so literally marked the first step in not only the physical healing process, but mentally as well. I recognized that I was still alive for a reason. I don't know what that reason is, but I'm not going to waste the opportunity I've been given. Second chances give you the opportunity to be more aware of how to impact the lives of other people – even if it is in some small act of kindness like holding the elevator, helping someone with their suitcase, or maybe just thanking someone for doing their job with a little extra effort.

No one knows when something as life altering as a major illness is going to tap you on the shoulder and say: "It's your turn." When it does, an opportunity is created to look at all the ways you can get better. There is no healing power in feeling sorry for yourself or wondering "why me?" I recognized that part of getting better is to figure out how to employ all the mental, physical and spiritual resources you have to make the best of your situation.

Lying around in my hospital bed, I thought about this a lot and came up with the keys to healing for me. I looked for things that I had some control over beyond the procedures, evaluations and meds...I came up with the Five Fs –

- Family

- Faith

- Friends

- Fitness, and

- Fun.

Each one is an avenue to healing available each day to you and those around you. They are important not just as a patient, but for family, friends and caregivers. Even if right now you can clearly identify only one of these as a positive source from which to draw strength, you can use it to get better and, maybe, incorporate some of the others over time.

In the pages to come, we'll look at each of the Five "Fs" and discuss the role of each one in the healing process. Here's a snapshot:

Family: We'll examine the function (and dysfunction), as well as the presence (or lack thereof) of family and how it impacts the healing process. We'll look at the challenges and the potential that exists with family being present and proactive. And, we'll look at how to connect (or reconnect). We'll also talk to the family members who are reading this book to let them know the importance of their role in the healing process for a loved one. There are lessons to be learned for all involved with the goal of getting the patient back to some semblance of their old functional (or dysfunctional) self.

Faith: We'll look at the importance of Faith, but my goal is not to push my religion on anyone or pontificate about what you should do. Mostly, I'll take you through the journey I am on trying to understand what is, for me, a very complicated part of the healing process. God's plan can be perplexing. It's difficult to put your situation into perspective. So many people say, "I'll be praying for you." I always took that with a grain of salt until I felt, firsthand, how powerful prayer can be – whether you are the one doing it or others are praying for you. Faith is belief in a source higher than yourself. If you, like me, have believed that you've always been able to beat the odds – to win despite the circumstances, where will you turn when your personal well runs dry? God can be your strongest ally in the healing process. This can be a time of reinforcing and growing your own relationship with God, but only if you open yourself up to it.

Friends: Bette Midler once sang about how you've "gotta have friends." Friends play a different role than family. Your relationship and dialogue with them isn't the same as you have with family members. You ask for, and need, different things from friends, and rely on them in varying ways. The context of your friendships – neighbors, church, school, sports, business - also determines how best they can help in your healing. Friends have an opportunity to really brighten your day and help you to feel better. I'm going to introduce you to some of my friends and how our relationship has evolved during my illness.

Fitness: For me, this involved both mental and physical fitness. Each is an essential piece in the getting better puzzle. You and your doctors have to work together to decide how you physically heal, but your mind is the engine behind it all. Mentally, you have to prepare not only yourself, but those around you, for what's happening and for what is going to happen next. Maybe it's just getting into the right mindset for surgery, the ongoing treatment plans or rehab. At the onset of my illness, it was coming to grips with the fact that I had an incurable disease and dealing with the possibility that I might not be here as long as I had imagined. It's hard to get your head around that until you're in that situation. Another part of the mental fitness routine is to prepare for the conversations that you will inevitably have with family and friends. They may be having a tough time with the mental game as well.

Physically, you may be faced with many challenges, so it comes back to setting milestones for accomplishing something on each step of the healing journey. We need to be as strong as we can, both mentally and physically to handle adversity. Focusing on the physical activity that you can do versus what you can't do – and then doing it – is one of the keys to physically getting better.

Fun: Remember it's OK to be not-so-serious during this serious time. You don't have to be a comedian constantly looking for laughs – just find ways to lighten the mood. Fun can mean a lot of things, but it all starts with being friendly. Smiles are contagious and laughs can perk up everyone's day. As you read through these pages, you'll see how Fun weaves itself into a lot of the other areas. There's not really a separate section for Fun. It sort of resides in every chapter. We'll talk about how fun comes in many different forms and can help shape your healing environment.

My arduous climb to get out of the Grand Canyon is much like the long journey from initial symptoms to recovery. Family and friends can help push you through the steep parts. Faith can give you the strength, confidence and courage to take on the challenge. Fitness can prepare you mentally and physically to make it to the next milestone. And fun, when the opportunity presents itself, makes the journey more pleasant for you and all those around you. There's a message in these pages for all those involved in getting better: patients, family, friends and caregivers. Find the pieces of the puzzle that fit for you and put them to work.

FAMILY

Everyone in the Intensive Care Unit is wrestling with some sort of life threatening situation, so that means things weren't all that good for me either. I found myself asking: "What am I doing up here?" Was I really that sick? And, to top it off, my room was at the end of the hall, which created a gauntlet of sick folks for visitors to navigate through on their way to visit me.

None of that deterred the Landiak Parade – For much of the last 2+ decades, we traveled everywhere as a family: wife, Barbara; oldest son Nicholas; backpacker Elise; younger daughter, Olivia; son, Luke; and of course, dad. I knew that none of the visitation rules would keep them away from coming as a pack when they could. And thankfully, no one tried to confine them to specific hours or the "two at a time" rule. I think the nurses "get it" that family helps with the healing, so they allowed us to bend the rules a bit. (Thanks for that by the way). There was no way the four kids would have come without each other if they were all able to come as a team. They are incredibly close to one another despite being four diverse individuals and act as their own support team. They seem to draw strength from one another as much as I draw strength from them.

Coming to see me gave the kids their first true understanding of how serious my situation really was. This was a huge communication error on my part. In the 11 months between the canyon incident and my collapse at the racquetball court,

I had never really shared with them the severity of what was going on. They had an idea that my condition was serious, but I left them in limbo, holding my discomfort inside. As it turned out, even I didn't know how serious my situation was I until my collapse. Prior to the hospital, things seemed somewhat normal to them. Dad was at the dinner table, laughing, having a good time. I looked swollen and sick, but really tried to hide my symptoms, or so I thought. Plus, the doctors didn't know exactly why I was having so many problems. Dad was not on his back in a hospital bed up to that point. My daughter Olivia told my friend Dan that *"Dad and hospital beds— the two just didn't go together."*

When I was admitted to the hospital, I spent some time preparing myself for how to handle the first visit from the kids. One of the first things I was conscious of was that they would be looking at me in a way they'd never seen me before. What kind of first impression did I want to create? What picture did I want them to walk away with after visiting their Dad? I didn't want them to be scared walking in or out of the room. They were scared enough when they heard Dad almost died and was in the hospital. There's going to be something going on in each of their heads, so I had to think about each one and what they need from me to get through this in the best way possible. This is an important point – what do each of your family members need <u>from you</u> during this time?

It was great for me when they would come to the hospital. But there was more. I was confronted with the startling reality that any day in the last 18 months could have been the last time I saw them. And the same was true for them. I am so grateful to have a second chance – an opportunity to see each one of them, hug them and tell them that I love them every chance I get. They probably get tired of me wanting to give them big hugs all the time, but every hug is precious to me.

So when they showed up to see me in the hospital the first time, I greeted them with big smiles and made it a point to tell them how much I love them. (Note to family and close friends: smiles, hugs and kisses are great therapy). So, when they'd show up, I was waiting with a hug and a kiss, trying to keep it light. I'd put a smile on and tell them: "Dad's doing really well, beating all the doc's expectations." And, I was, by simply by being conscious.

After my collapse, I didn't sugar coat things – it's hard to when your heart monitor alarm is continually beeping in the background and nurses are constantly checking in to see if you went "Code Blue" on them. I'd provide a short answer to the "how you doin' dad?" question and then move on. "Luke, how's water polo? Nicholas, Elise, how's work? Olivia, how's school?" Sure, there were emotions. There weren't many tears in front of me, but I could see and feel their concern. At times, they looked scared. One of my big mistakes was not communicating what was going on every step of the way. At first, I thought holding back was the right thing to do…to protect them. Later, they told me that it raised, rather than reduced anxiety. I guess the natural inclination of any father is to protect his family. I wanted to shelter them from the breadth of the situation. In retrospect, I should have been up front with what was going on.

My efforts to keep things light with them meant a joke or two (or six), sometimes even at their expense. Joking around helps them all know I'm getting back on my game. It's important for me to bust their chops and for them to know that I can. And, by the way, I want them to know it's OK for them to bust my chops right back. One time, Luke stopped by after school and needed to use the bathroom in my room. He pops his head out and says, "Dad, there's a giant jug of pee in there." I realized the nurse who's supposed to measure my urine output (an odd and uncomfortable exercise) forgot to empty the bottle during her last visit. So I said to my son: "Luke, use the bottle. Pee in the bottle, then I'll make a contribution and when the nurse comes in to check, the whole thing will be full." Next thing you know, we've got this voluminous amount of liquid in the container.

The nurse comes by soon after. I start telling her that I've got to stop drinking so much water. "Check the bottle, you'll see."

She goes, "Oh, lord, that's the most I've ever seen." I keep up the scam, saying the docs told me to drink lots of water, but now she starts telling me that I should slow down so I don't wash all the medicine out of my system. As she starts pouring out this voluminous amount of liquid into the toilet, Luke and I started laughing really hard. She was unsure whether to record some or all of it, which has got to be two to three times what a normal fill up will be. She came out looking rather stunned. "When you got to go, you've got to go," I laughed. Eventually we told her what we did. She said something like: "I should've considered the source." I was hoping she'd say it was a world record. But, because of the meds I was on, I'd have failed the drug test, anyway.

I also had to understand that the kids had to go on with their lives. Work, school and activities added to the sense of normalcy. And still, they made it a point to get by often.

Barbara, always the straight man to my silly antics, was by my side almost all of the time in the hospital. Just the comfort of having her there was a big help. We talked about my medical condition some, but not as much as we talked about other stuff. I didn't want to talk about how poorly I felt or what was going to happen next. She saw all the monitors and, while she probably didn't know what some of them meant, she knew it wasn't good that they were always going off causing nurses to come running in. She would rarely say anything about that. She holds her innermost thoughts close to the vest. The doctors would come in to give a frank assessment of things and she'd ask really good questions. By the way, it's fine for family members to ask tough questions as well. Sometimes the patient isn't thinking as clearly as he/she should and it's nice to have someone to advocate for you. Barb didn't comment on the severity of the situation. Perhaps she didn't want to burden me with her reaction. I slept a lot. Opening my eyes to find her there was a huge comfort to me. Even if we didn't have anything to say, making eye contact and holding hands conveyed the message loud and clear.

So I guess the moral to this story is to let your family know what's going on. Encourage them to ask the doctors and nurses questions. And, let them know how much you appreciate the fact that they are there.

PICKING NUTS OFF THE
FAMILY TREE

Almost everything about my approach to healing can be traced back to family. I guess I was a lucky kid. My Dad gave me a tremendous work ethic and a desire to outperform his expectations. My mom offered plenty of support and encouragement. As I got older and into high school, she always knew I could do it, no matter what "it" was at that moment.

As the youngest of three children, I spent the majority of my formative years in State College, Pennsylvania. We moved there from New Jersey when I was in 7th grade.

Dad worked as an engineer for Penn State University, which offered a lifestyle change for him and us. He had spent 25 years at sea working on different ships, but mostly on the S.S. United States passenger liner. I didn't see him a lot during my early years. He'd come home after two or sometimes three weeks at sea and not really have any fun. He was a serious guy and never had much playtime with his kids due to the amount of travel and long list of "To Do's" he'd assign himself when he was home. Maybe the reason I'm so not serious is because he was serious enough for the both of us. I'd be sarcastic with him, tell a joke, and he wouldn't see the humor. It never dawned on me that maybe I just wasn't as funny as I thought. Mom, however, would usually humor me with an obligatory chuckle, then give me some sage advice like: "don't annoy your father." Still the lesson of laughter remained. It can serve us well during a very stressful times. Maybe it can work for you in your situation. It couldn't hurt…except when someone told me a joke that made me laugh really hard right after my open heart surgery. That actually did hurt.

My dad approached challenges with a "to do" list mentality that came from being a world class marine engineer. He could figure out and fix anything. As a youngster, I had to be right by his side, handing him wrenches and hammers and getting out of the way when things would start flying around and fingers got smashed. That's when the colorful language dad acquired at sea would also start to fly. Learning new vocabulary was great fun for a young apprentice. Unfortunately for me, my mom was ready with a bar of soap if I decided to try out any of my newly learned vocabulary in the neighborhood.

Above everything else was the lawn. It had to be perfect. He'd have me cut the grass two times a week with a hand mower because it did a better job than a gas powered model. All of that youthful grass cutting experience has led me to have the worst lawn in my neighborhood these days – a fact I am very proud of, by the way. Every time I see how crappy my lawn looks, I think of how much extra time it gave me to be with my kids and to be a dad. Oh, and I don't fix <u>anything</u>. Fortunately, I do know how to operate a phone to call people who have the ability and desire to fix stuff in one tenth of the time it would take for me to do it myself…and all I have to do is pay them. Is this a great country or what? That's why we go to doctors. Left to my own devices, I nearly killed myself with a big bowl of denial topped with poor judgment sauce.

LESSONS FROM THE
FAM: MOM & DAD

Almost everyone who is sick can draw from their own life experiences and use them to get better. As I laid in bed, one of the exercises I did was to think about the traits of each one of my family members and how that might help me to improve. My work ethic developed from seeing how hard my dad worked, a characteristic of the Greatest Generation. I was lucky to have my dad around through my high school and college years. I think we really became closest when I went to college. He worked at Penn State and I fell in love with the place and decided to go to school there. I'd meet him for lunch between classes and we'd talk about everything and nothing in particular. He'd take me to Roy Roger's for a burger or a roast beef sandwich. Back in Jr. High and High School, dad would say: "we're leaving in 45 minutes, go cut the lawn." (with the hand mower). The old boy always had me running like that. Maybe that was his way of keeping me out of trouble and at least it kept me in good shape. As a kid, I always worked hard, whether it was delivering papers for a nickel apiece, shoveling snow for $5 a driveway or cutting our grass for nothing. I think all of that led me to start my own company 25 years ago. I run a training and consulting firm that specializes in the areas of sales, customer service and the management of those functions. We help companies grow their sales and improve their profitability. Like my dad, I travelled a lot as well. This was never in my plan. It just worked out that way and gave me a greater appreciation for my dad who did what he had to do to provide for his family. I ended up doing the same thing. Up until recently, he'd wake up early every morning and do his exercises, then make breakfast for my mom. Most days, he'll get out for a short walk, and at 93, he still played golf. Now he is 95 and recovering from heart surgery and a slew of post-operative complications, but he still gets around. He's truly an inspiration for me.

The launch of this book got delayed by my dad getting ill. He had always been in great shape for his age, then one day I noticed a big change in his breathing. The doctor told him that his Aortic valve needed to be replaced and on top of that, they later found that he also needed a triple bypass. His choices were to do nothing and live for 3-6 months, or have surgery. He was deemed strong enough to undergo open heart surgery at age 94 to replace a valve and perform the triple bypass. This is something they won't even consider attempting on most people his age, but dad is a tough guy who was in amazing shape for his age. The surgery went well, but he had to fight through 3 ½ months of post-operative complications and we thought we were going to lose him several times. He was in and out of the hospital 3 times for a total of 46 days over a 70-day period. During this time and right up to today, my role was switched from patient to caregiver. Looking at the healing process from the foot of the bed with someone else as the focus has been illuminating. Now, I have a better understanding of what my family was going through. Moreover, I had to put my own process to work with someone else…someone I loved who might be dying. There's a big difference between what you do as a patient and what you do as a caregiver. That said, the 5 F's still apply. However, the application of them is entirely different. In the caregiver role, I drive him to rehab and doctor's appointments and manage a lot of the medical details for him. These are things any family member could pitch in to do. My sisters live far away, but coordinate trips in to be with the folks and take care of things while I'm travelling or just taking a break from my duties with dad and mom. They offer a different brand of caregiving that mom and dad really appreciate. I think just their presence helps. We'll discuss the importance of "being there" in just a moment.

My mom has a good sense of humor and I could always make her laugh. I think that's why I got away with a lot growing up as a kid. She's a pretty amazing lady. Now 95, I sometimes think she's healthier than I am, which is remarkable when you consider she had a huge stroke not too long ago that was followed, a short time later, by a bout with lymphoma and then a melanoma that was cancerous and had to be removed. Most recently, she had a fall and broke 3 ribs, but rarely complained and recovered remarkably fast. Time has taken it's toll on some of her faculties, and she is suffering from short-term memory loss. She's surprisingly matter of fact about her situation. I don't think she ever missed a rehab session after her stroke. My dad is the same way. It is that type of discipline and consistency that serve as a good example for me. If my 90+ year old parents can do it, what excuse do I have? They walk daily when the weather allows and dad is religious about his daily exercises. Now I can use all of these life experiences with my mom and dad as the foundation and inspiration for improving my health. It's like another place from which to draw healing strength. When I get lazy and don't want to do my own rehab routine, I can think of mom and dad. They are a part of my inspiration every day. What's yours?

JUST SHOW UP

My two sisters – Karen, who's nine years older, and Marilyn, five years older – and I didn't have much time to connect as kids, although their motherly instincts did try to take over at times when I was younger. We would be together at mandatory family dinners or be jammed together in the back seat of the Buick along with a big red Coleman™ cooler during vacations, but we didn't have the type of strong bond growing up like the one my kids have. We became closer as the years grew on and we started having families. Even so, both became really concerned when I started to go through all of this, and each has come through to help me in her own way. Marilyn does medical litigation research. She probably should have been a doctor. She's plenty smart and likes to act the part when conversing with all the medical types. She has a knack for deciphering medical mumbo jumbo (a technical term encompassing all things health related that regular people can't understand). Maybe my next book will be a translation book. Just like another foreign language, I would convert medical terms like "stenosis" to terms that patients can actually understand like "getting smaller or more narrow." Of course, she wanted to know what I had, do some research and then send me all sorts of information about what she found. She'd also give me suggestions about what to ask the doctors. After the misdiagnosis phase ended and I was told I had sarcoidosis, she read up on that too. It got her pretty worried because it's pretty nasty stuff, and she sent me info on that as well to help me understand better what's going on inside me. At the very least, it gave me additional questions to ask my docs.

If you're a relative or friend and have the ability to help one of us patients to translate doctor-speak into plain terms that an average person can understand, feel free to ask if you can help.

My sister Karen is retired, but was one of the greatest elementary school teachers of all time. A product of the 60's, she's still to this day all full of peace and love…and she too, loves her little brother. After my vacation in the ICU, Karen, who lives in New York, was getting ready for a trip to Ireland. She calls me up to say she's coming to visit. "Great," I said. "When?" Her reply: "Tomorrow." I said, "But you're going to Ireland in three days." She spent 13 hours on the train that night, visited me for five hours and then spent another 13 hours to get home to finish packing before rushing off to Ireland. (She's a full-blooded Ukrainian, but thinks she's Irish). She wanted her last hug, I guess. I even said that to her. "What, you think I'm not going to be here when you get back?" She didn't answer. I think she just thought I was going to pass away while she was in some pub having a Guinness. Karen's rules to live by include one very simple idea: "Just show up." It's a pretty good rule, actually. If you're a relative trying to decide whether to go see your kin in the hospital or whether you should drop in for a visit at home during their recovery, take my sister's advice and just show up. You can also show up by making a phone call, sending an email, doing some research and sending a link to an article or just dropping a card in the mail. Several of my friends told me that they didn't call because they didn't want to bother me, but when we reconnected, it was great.

Flowers are nice, but your face or voice is the best – and, if you're going to show up, you might want to call first to let the patient know you're coming to make sure they're in a condition to receive company …and bring some cookies.

When I had my more recent open heart surgery, my sisters devised a plan. Marilyn would be in Pennsylvania with my parents, who didn't need the stress of travelling added to the stress of their son getting operated on. Karen would catch a flight and stay with us to keep the folks back in PA informed of what was going on. It was a good plan and a great example of family involved in the healing and helping process. I didn't have to worry about my mom and dad and they could worry less about me.

TAKE MY WIFE...PLEASE.

Henny Youngman was a comedian in the 40's, 50's and 60's who started out many of his routines with this line. He was known as the king of the one-liner. He'd lampoon their relationship, but there was no doubt he loved this woman and she was his partner through it all. If you never had the pleasure of seeing this man perform, I heartily recommend going on YouTube and checking him out. And, he does a lot of medical jokes that might give you a chuckle.

I met the most important woman in my life, my wife Barbara, as a freshman at Penn State. On the second day of English class, this gal – (a total knockout by the way), transfers into the class and walks in late. (That should have told me something right away because to this day, she is perpetually late for everything – and yes, I am going to pay dearly for publishing that comment).

So, my friend and I were seated in the very front row and as soon as I see her, I immediately tell him: "I got dibs." So the next day I got there early and moved from my studious front row seat to the back row to sit down next to her and strike up a conversation. This gives you an idea of my collegiate priorities. Another guy walks in and says I took his seat. I said, "You've got a new seat. This is college, man, there are no assigned seats. Go sit over there." I didn't care where he went. I just wanted him to go away so I could sit beside this great looking gal who probably thought I was a bit nuts. In a way, I guess I was, and she would likely tell you that I still am.

Since I lived in town and had a car, I offered her a ride back to her dorm. She agreed, and we proceeded to walk about a mile completely across campus to get my car. I opened her door and then drove back the way we came, past the building about a quarter mile to her room. We could have walked to her dorm in one quarter of the time, but it was a nice day and for some reason, she decided to join me. We didn't date right away because she was still with her high school boyfriend, but we still hung out. I always invited her to do things. She eventually saw the light. Thirty-five years and multiple moves around the country later, here we are...in this situation that always happened to other people and wasn't supposed to happen to us. But here we are and I'm lucky to have someone who cares so much and understands. Many times, a lot goes unspoken... just having people you love nearby provides the comfort and support necessary to help with feeling better. When one partner is sick, his or her partner goes through their own anguish and it can take its toll both mentally and physically. Frankly, I don't know what I would do if she wasn't here. If Getting Better is about more than recovering from illness, than oddly enough, through all this, in some ways our relationship might also be getting better.

HEALING LESSONS FROM THE KIDS

As I mentioned earlier, I have 4 kids. For Barbara and I, they are the center of our lives. During my illness, I found that I could draw strength from the things I admired in other people. From each one of my kids for instance, I thought about their positive attributes and how to draw strength and motivation to get better. If you have kids, nieces, nephews, grandchildren or godchildren, they can be inspiring and even therapeutic. They can make you laugh. They can make you think. They can give you reasons to push forward. Almost everyone knows someone who went through tremendous difficulty and somehow persevered. I want my kids to be proud of their dad, regardless of what ultimately happens or how things go down the road. This helps with the mental elements of getting through difficult periods. Think about how one or more of the young people in your life might help you with the healing process. If not, maybe you have a brother, sister, or other relative, best friend or even another patient from whom you can draw inspiration. I laid in my hospital bed one night and gave some thought to some of the things I appreciate most about my kids and could draw upon to get through my own ordeal. Each have characteristics that help me with the process of getting better.

DETERMINATION

To beat an illness or recover from one, you have to have a high level of determination.

Luke is my youngest. He is an amazingly accomplished young man and I'm so proud of him. When I first got home from the hospital, I couldn't work for some time, so I got to be with him a lot during his high school years before he left for college. Luke and I have a special bond that goes back to his grade school days when I was his soccer coach. After I got sick, I would still go to his sporting events. He would look up in the stands and when we made eye contact, it was a reminder for me that I need to press forward. For both of us (or at least for me), this momentary connection was really important. I think he gets that I was in the stands to support him - win, lose or draw. But he also knew that he almost lost his dad. Every time in the last couple years when I got to one of his events felt like a bonus. Regardless of how poorly I felt, I went. It helped me feel better and wasn't something that I would take for granted. I'm so happy to have had the opportunity to see him compete, even now, because he gives it his all and works so hard to win. In the healing process, it's important to have the same type of determination to do what's necessary to get better. I can feel Luke saying to me, "You can beat this." For me, that type of support is really important. I can think back on his events and draw strength from his determination to win. Now I want him to see me giving my all to live as best I can, have fun and work to get better. I don't want to let him down, so I'm trying to beat this thing with every fiber of my being. I feel like I have to make it through the day to be there for him and wake up to make him breakfast or see him do his thing. Whether it's on a field, in a pool, on a wrestling mat, on a stage or in a classroom, he wants to win. I latch on to that and think about it a lot. It's an important part of my healing process. Sometimes healing is hard. We have to be determined to do the things that will help us improve. He has a mantra that he uses frequently and semi-jokingly in a wide variety of settings, but every time I feel like I'm up against the wall, I replay his voice in my head and hear him say: "You gotta want it, dad!"

FIND THE JOY

When you are well, you can find joy in a lot of different places, but when you're really sick and facing some serious problems head on, there are times when it can seem downright impossible.

My Olivia laughs and smiles her way through life in a spontaneous response to the world with a manner that forces you to smile along with her. At any moment, she will break out in dance in the kitchen, humming along to the song of the week or one that she just made up, or bust out some hip hop moves and then look at you like: "Did you see that?" She's got such an unbelievable spirit. All I have to do is think about my redhead and I smile. When she went off to college, I missed her something awful. She came home a lot and just having her around made me "feel" better. To this day, when she is around, I hug her as many times per day as she will allow. It probably drives her crazy, but she humors me. It revives me. Olly, and people like her, can help you find the joy in life. They are rare and moments with them are to be treasured. I'm convinced that being with people who have this gift is therapeutic. That's Olly. She's beautiful inside and out…an amazing human being. Of course, she has her moments when things get her down as well, but she pushes through it. Here's the thing: If you're a caregiver, find a way to spread joy around as a way to help the patient (and everyone else) feel a little better. Patients can do the same thing by surprising people with a positive outlook on life, despite life-threatening circumstances. If I ever start to lose perspective or feel sorry for myself over my situation, I just think of Olivia dancing in the kitchen or belting out a tune and I can't help but smile and get my head back on track. She's taught me to find the joy – even when I have to look a little harder for it at times. Oh, and she gives the best back rubs in the universe.

CONFIDENCE

Building up the confidence to deal with whatever comes at you as a patient or a caregiver is something you have to consciously and continuously think about and work on.

My daughter Elise and I are very similar because she keeps her wits about her when things get dicey. And, she doesn't back down from challenges like lugging Dad out of the Grand Canyon or taking on a company that she thinks ripped her off. Her incredibly strong will and her unwillingness to back down remind me to be confident in my ability to get better. When she was growing up, we would sometimes mix it up because she can be bullheaded about things...me too, I guess. But, that can work in your favor too. Sometimes, you just need to pick your head up and face the situation (whether you're the patient or family member) head on. And, she has an ability to boil it down and tell it like it is. She gets annoyed when I don't communicate. I think she just wants to feel like everything is going to work out and that dad is going to be fine...but, she wants to know what's going on. She got married during my illness and I was so grateful to be there to walk her up the aisle, something I wasn't sure that I'd be around to do. We were in the back of the church ready to walk up the aisle to the altar. I figured I'd go console her and tell her not to be nervous, but she spoke first and hit me with "I love you daddy." On came the faucets and I started crying like the emotional wreck that I vowed not to be. The wedding party had almost all taken arms and strolled up the aisle. The coordinator looks at us and says: "10 seconds." With 5 seconds to lift off, Elise grabs my arm, looks me straight in the eyes and says: "Pull it together dad!" She was as cool as a cucumber. That's the kind of confidence you need going into a procedure or test or when getting news from your doctor. I can still hear her say: "Pull it together dad." Somehow I managed and it was a magical moment. Right before we took the first step, she asks: "Ready?" I said, "yes." We smiled at each other and off we went both utterly confident that it was going to be great…and it was. I'll never forget that moment.

Even though our last trip to the Canyon was almost my last trip anywhere, I wouldn't trade it for anything. Our trips there are special memories. I can remember her self-assuredness when flirting near the edge to get a better view and powering up the steep inclines with one goal in mind. I think there is no doubt in her mind that dad is going to come through this and be fine some day, and that kind of confidence is very reassuring. I sometimes have to take a moment and calm myself before any sticky medical situation I'm going into. So, now I just say to myself: "Pull it together dad."

CARPE' DIEM

My oldest, Nicholas, could easily be on one of those survival adventure shows. He's the rugged, outdoorsman type with a great head on his shoulders and a penchant for getting the most out of every experience. He watches his diet, is a cross-fit trainer and focuses on getting better in most every aspect of his life...and on helping other people do the same. He reminds me that we need to seize the moments as they present themselves and take the opportunities to enjoy the people, places and things around us. To that end, he recently returned from mountain climbing on Mont Blanc in France. Why? Because a friend invited him and it seemed like a good idea at the time. When I was his age, I was like that – perhaps a bit more rebellious, but like that nonetheless. One of the many good times we have shared together was an adventure vacation in New Zealand. It was truly one of those phenomenal moments in life that you can look back on and say, "Remember when we went river surfing? jumped out of a perfectly good airplane? went skin diving in one of the most beautiful places on earth? got chased by a bighorn sheep in the mountains?" Nicholas and I are really close and always have been. In my days of running around the country nonstop for work, I made it a habit to always take the last flight out so I could coach the kids in soccer or make it to their school or sporting events. I remember when Nicholas wrestled in middle school, I'd often have to leave before the meets ended. He would spot me when I'd point to my watch and get up to leave, and he'd walk across the entire gym to make sure he gave me – in front of everyone — a hug and a kiss goodbye. What middle school kid does that? -Especially a son to his dad. He did it all through high school and still does it to this day. Luke does the same thing. People with the type of heart Nicholas shows can help us all understand that we must make the most of the moments we have with those that we care about. He certainly makes the most of each opportunity and does a great job caring about the people around him. He reminds me to be a caring person and try to find something to do within my capabilities that I can look back on at the end of the day and think: I accomplished this today. He is also very devout in his faith and reminds me to be thankful for each day and the opportunities that present themselves.

So those are my kids. I am so blessed that they love their dad and share bits of their lives with me…and let me share some of my life with them. Think about the people you care about and what you appreciate in them. Identify the qualities you admire and what they can do to help you heal. It works in reverse too. If you are the relative or friend of someone who is sick, know that they look to you for your support, your encouragement and your hugs. There may be something about you that they can draw strength or comfort or inspiration from. Patients can provide the same for the people that care about them. Everyone has something positive to offer. Offer it. Think about the people from whom you can draw inspiration and make them a part of your getting better process.

FAMILY, FRIENDS AND STRANGERS WANTED

We've lived and raised our kids in Naperville, Illinois, since 1989. Throughout my life – and more so now – my wife and kids have had the most profound impact on me. You probably got that. They've changed my world view from all about me to all about them. Since taking ill, every moment is even more meaningful. When I was in the hospital the first time, I had a lot of time to think about how much each one means to me and how they help me to heal. Maybe you have relatives and friends that can do the same for you. I dip into this well a lot… and pull what I need to get me out of bed in the morning and through the challenges of each new day. Who in your life can make you stronger, help you to cope and help you to heal? I'm fortunate to have a strong family support team behind me, but it doesn't have to be a family member. It could be a close friend, a new acquaintance, one of the patients you've met who is going through a similar situation, or even someone you can chat with on-line in a support website for people with your disease. The key is to find someone you can talk to.

If you are on the healthy end of the relationship, be part of your patient's support team. Don't know where to start? Just show up.

YOU'VE GOT TO HAVE FRIENDS

Throughout life we make friends that come from different places. Maybe you've got church friends, people you went to school with, drinking buddies, a friend you hit the mall with, someone you play cards or sports with, or any number of other activities that match your lifestyle. There's no doubt that friends can help you get better, and consider all the different types of friends you have on your side. I have Faith friends: Father Pat, Deacon Joe and others I have connected with spiritually. There are my soccer teammates. Of course, I have my locked-in crew of longtime friends and fraternity brothers who always have had my back. There are the neighbors and friends you met as your kids grew up with theirs. And, when I started to think about my business, I took stock in my "work" friends that I could turn to. What didn't strike me immediately was the onetime friends you can make in the hospital, fellow patients that you might never see again, but can stay in your memory forever. Throughout the book, we'll talk about how important friends are in the healing process and some of them can be just like family. It's important to stay in touch and keep your friends informed as best you can, lest you fall victim to disease fatigue. Once you are out of the hospital and on the mend, it can easily be assumed that you are "better" even if you are still very sick and your road to recovery is just beginning. Disease fatigue sets in when you are sick for a long time and people assume you are better or get distracted by other happenings in their lives. Don't get discouraged. This is quite normal. Time between visits and calls go from days to weeks to months. I've learned that it is up to me to keep in touch with friends. Some friends are always there, but most people have their own lives to live and can get occupied with other things. This is just the way it is. The internet is an amazing tool. Online support groups provide you with a group of people who can understand what you are going through as, unfortunately, many are sick as well. It's hard to feel sorry for yourself when there are other people who are worse off than you. Internet support group friends are always there. You might not ever meet them, but they like having other people to talk with. I make it a habit to be upbeat and understanding, and try not to commiserate about negatives.

NOTE TO FRIENDS: JUST SHOW UP

Friends have a different role in the healing process, mainly because, unlike family, there's a different connection. Family is there because they love you and/or, in some instances, because they feel obligated – not in a bad way – to be beside you in the hospital. Friends, on the other hand, can come and go as they please. They might have a sense of duty or loyalty to visit you in the hospital, but could be delayed or tied up in the apprehension some people get when they think about going into that environment. This is where my older sister, Karen's "Just Show Up" rule really comes in handy. It takes all the thinking out of the equation. If the person in the hospital is important to you, just show up to lend your support. Figure out something you can bring to brighten their day – a story, joke, book, magazine article, game or anything that might help with their healing. When you think about it, that is a great rule, isn't it?

Some time back, the wife of a soccer friend passed away suddenly. The guys on the team talked about going, but no one really made plans. A group of us got together and decided to go to the funeral. Our friend was so appreciative that we showed up. It truly makes a difference. The Just Show Up rule works when people are hurting or healing. It gives an opportunity for the patient to communicate to their friends that what they do – even just stopping by – makes them feel better for that moment and helps the healing process.

It's funny how, as we grow up, at all the different stages in life, we are willing to say just about anything to our closest friends. In my group of close friends, we've said some pretty ridiculous things to one another to make each other laugh. We've also shared some serious conversations about those situations in life that are hard to talk about. Think about how you interact with your variety of friends. Who do you confide in? Which one can you watch a game with and, without a second thought, shout at the TV with? When illness or tragedy happens, so many people don't tell their friends what they need. And, if those friends are apprehensive about approaching you, it could lead to some moments of confusion where the patient wonders: "Where's so and so? Why hasn't he/she called?" There were a couple of guys who I wondered about. One in particular said he didn't know what I was going through. Sometimes that's the case. They just don't know about your situation. I got an email from a friend's wife that she sent out to a large group of folks telling about her husband's illness. It gave us all a chance to respond.

While in the hospital, I dropped a note to my longtime friend, Mike Murphy to update him on my condition. He immediately responded to say he'd be in town for business the following week, but didn't know if I wanted the company because of how I might be feeling. This is a common sentiment among friends that prevents them from coming to see you. Murph, well, he just showed up, and my entire family happened to be there. Murph is one of those rare people who are both genuinely friendly and naturally funny. He could have easily been a stand-up comedian or certainly a comedy writer. He made us all laugh. His presence lightened the atmosphere and made everyone feel better. At one point he launched into a monologue about my crisis as merely a means to get attention. We all laughed and I nearly busted my stitches as he continued to lampoon me. Here's the thing. If he didn't know I was in trouble, he wouldn't have made the offer and my family and I would have missed a great opportunity to feel better – at least for that moment. Since then, he's been in town again and one time a while back, he stopped by to join me on a walk around the neighborhood. It happened to be a couple days after I had received some news that my condition had deteriorated. He couldn't have come at a better time. After covering the latest bad news, we were back to yucking it up and he had me smiling again. People like Murph make you really appreciate the time they make for you and it can open the door to an even stronger relationship.

You can and should put out the feelers to friends to let them know it's OK to stop by, to send a funny card or just do whatever they would like as a way to help you through the healing process. When you're back home, breakfasts and lunches with friends can work. Man, it meant so much when my soccer buddy Tony came into the hospital with a ball and said, "This is the ball we're going to use the first game you're back." Soccer pals Ted, Paul, Gary and Mike also dropped by to keep me company and shuffle around the floor with me. That's something that I appreciated more than they know.

Also during my hospital stay, my longtime co-worker and friend Meg, who has been with my company since the beginning, brought me her special oatmeal raisin cookies – my absolute favorite. You won't find the cookie lady at Costco handing these babies out. She makes the best. I probably wasn't supposed to have them while in the hospital, but I'd sneak one out of the container every so often and fire it down. Meg's young daughter, the cutest little creature in the world, can always put a smile on my face. She tagged along as well and when there's a little kid around just being a little kid, it can be fun as long as they don't accidently yank out your IV.

My soccer pal Ted was one of the big surprises. He came to the hospital, brought me a book and showed me pictures of his new house in Colorado. Ted has a very dry sense of humor-so much so, that you don't know if what he just said was meant to be funny. But he is very sincere and he cares. Ted would walk up and down the halls with me, talk about soccer and his new house. He's just a good guy. I learned more about Ted in those visits than in all the years we played soccer. Our relationship grew because he decided to show up for several shuffles with me at the hospital and even rode his oversized bike to my house a few times. A past co-worker, Michelle, who had dropped off a book on the FBI, called to check up on me. She has this big, wonderfully bombastic voice – "HEY MARK, HOW'S IT GOING? JUST CHECKING UP ON YOU…" That's her, I'd be real disappointed if she wasn't herself. That's what we all want. You don't want friends to act differently because you are sick, unless, of course, they were jerks before. Michelle even came over to have lunch with me after I was discharged.

I'm fortunate to have these and other examples of how "showing up" takes on many shapes and sizes. You know your friends pretty well, so there's nothing wrong with helping them understand what they can do to aid you in getting better.

If you're the friend, and you know and care about a person in need, think: "What can I do to help this person get better?" It's often the little things that make a big difference. The "in the neighborhood and wanted to stop by," the thoughtful card or email, the book or movie, a meal for the family, all make a difference. So, when in doubt, just show up.

REMINDERS, ROUTINES AND PIEROGIS

Mental reminders from family and regular communication with friends can help motivate some patients in the daily push to get better. It was worse before, but my illness still prevents me from doing many of the things that I used to do, I take advantage of what I can as the opportunities present themselves. Sometimes that's just a conversation or simple act of kindness to someone you might not even know. Sometimes it's just trying to be a good example or listener for others going through trials in their lives. And, sometimes it's just getting out of bed in the morning and getting the day started when you feel like just laying there.

People always tell Barbara and I that we have great kids. I think that a lot myself. I certainly appreciate what my wife's been able to do. She's been the glue for us while I was travelling or distracted by work. Our kids have always been, and will always be Number One in her world. Being sick and working less means I'm around the house more. It's now I see the things she does and how hard she works, to keep our household going. And I thought being around the house all the time might create some problems. Admittedly, I can be a pain in the ass – I couldn't drive a car for almost a year, and to this day, have times when I'm unfit to be behind the wheel mostly because of my load of medications. That meant I ended up interrupting her day with requests to chauffer me here and there. I heard her telling someone that having me around all the time is fine, except when we're driving. She said I'm always telling her to look out for this guy or that driver. She's OK with that to a certain degree, then she gives me the "it's time for you to shut up or get out of the car" look. I guess I just need not be so observant.

What I am really paying attention to is everyday life. Nothing is routine anymore, certainly not the gathering around the dinner table. We've always eaten together as a family, a rarity in this day and age, so it's such a cool feeling to look around and see these young adults sitting in spots where they once occupied high chairs. When the kids were all at home, dinner together was always sacrosanct. When all four of the kids are there with Barbara and me, which is a rarity anymore, it's more of a celebration than anything else – at least for mom and dad.

Sunday breakfast is another thing – again with meals, did I mention I like to eat? – that is no longer mundane. I've made the big breakfast on Sunday forever. No matter how bad I feel from my meds, I'm making breakfast. My one area of culinary expertise is…eggs. It's gone from a weekly routine to something I derive so much pleasure out of regardless of which symptoms I happened to wake up with that day. These moments put me back into context for my family. I can appear more "normal."

And, yes, I do like to eat. Meds aren't a food group, but they can have a big impact on appetite. I was fortunate to be referred to rheumatologist Dr. Nadera Sweiss, a brilliant woman who is affiliated with the University of Illinois Medical Center in Chicago, to work with my cardiologists to sort out the best possible med plan and monitor the nasty side effects they can have.

At one appointment, I mentioned that I had put on 10 pounds and noticed some swelling in my stomach. I asked the doctor if my ravenous appetite and weight gain were due to the meds and, if so, what should I do? She looked me right in the eyes with a serious look and said matter-of-factly: "Stop eating so much." For those of you keeping score at home, that's $400 for an office visit to tell me to control my weight gain by eating less. Wow, why didn't I think of that? It seems some docs are worth their weight in piroghi's, and will kid around with you once they know you're receptive to that kind of sarcastic response. Add her to my list of favorite doctors, as well.

NURSES

I have a favorite list of nurses as well. In fact, my wife might tell you that I have a thing for nurses. I love the ones who go beyond the normal routine, seeing you as more than just another sick person in a bed. The special ones try to get to know about you as a person. There seems to be a lot of these people at Edward Hospital in Naperville, Illinois and Loyola Medical Center in Maywood, IL. They connect with you, laugh with you and some even pray with you. They're the ones who turn the other way when you've got some contraband oatmeal raisin cookies (thanks Meg), and then enjoy sharing one with you when no one is looking. These nurses think about what you need to heal and give you a little more of themselves to help you get there. They have the ability to brighten the room with an energy for their job that can become both contagious and therapeutic. I'll talk a lot about "my" nurses in these pages. I've listed as many as I can remember in the acknowledgements. If I missed one of you, please forgive me and chalk it up to the meds you gave me. I love you nonetheless. Let me introduce you to one of my nurses.

Sarah, fresh out of nursing school, couldn't have been more than 22 or so. Her enthusiasm for the job reminded me of a kid taking her first roller coaster ride. I had been in the hospital for about a week when Sarah first entered my room, and I looked like hell. They wouldn't let me take a shower to keep my surgical wound from getting wet, so I looked like the people on the TV show, "Naked and Alive," except I was in my hospital gown. Still, I felt like someone who hadn't shaved or showered for a week because I hadn't shaved or showered in a week. My hair looked like I had attempted to comb out my bed head with a pork chop. It just happened that Sarah's first encounter with me came on a day when I had once again scribbled my own "doctor's orders" on the treatment board. The following was this day's effort. Under the "real items" written by the last nurse on duty, I added my own personal recommendations in an effort to catch my nurses off guard.

Treatment for March 2nd

- *Magnesium Drip*

- *Vitals Every 2 Hours*

- *Replace IV*

- *Lab Work Per Doctor's Orders*

- *Sponge Bath and Massage*

- *Bowl of Fresh Grapes*

Can you guess which ones I added? Sure you can. Sarah read through the first four items, then burst out laughing, just as I had hoped. She checked out my blood pressure, heart rate, EKG and temp. I was a bit self-conscious about the road kill resting on my scalp, and then she asked if I'd like to wash my hair. "How can I do that? It's not supposed to get wet." I asked. Turns out, the hospital has this waterless shampoo that is inside a shower cap and only needs to be massaged into the hair. "Do you want me to get you one?" Sarah offered. She had me at waterless shampoo and, without missing a beat, I said, yes. When Sarah came back, she asked if I'd like her to do the shampoo. (This is the closest I'm going to get to a sponge bath and a massage, I thought to myself, so definitely go for it, Mark). "Yes, thank you. That would be very nice." She put the cap on and began a blissful scalp massage that created a Nirvana only known by those getting a hair and scalp massage after having been pent up in the hospital for a week and those who have actually been to Nirvana. "Oh, that's fantastic," I told her. No doubt about it, during the massage and for several hours afterward, I felt much, much better. As Sarah left, I thanked her profusely and she said, "No problem. We'll work on those grapes." Across the room, Barbara gave me "the look" and told me to wipe the gigantic grin off my face. "I hope you're not expecting me to massage your scalp when we get home. Maybe we should just shave your head." I gave her a look of disappointment and muttered, "Thanks, honey."

UNDERSTANDING AND COPING

While we are on the topic of massages…as I mentioned earlier, Olivia has the magic touch when it comes to the knots in my back that show up uninvited or the "buffalo hump" that the steroids can form on the back of my neck. It feels like I've got a rubber hose or something in there. Olivia can knock it out like no one's business. I'll just hold up my hands and rub my fingers together in a massaging motion, and she's right there with a neck massage without complaint. I've always been fortunate to have a family that's pretty much in tune with one another. We were that way before I got sick. It's become more apparent now, in different ways, like when someone offers a hand to me when I'm ready to stand up. They've seen me queasy and even fall, so they're at the ready. I med load on the weekends, so at church on Sundays, Luke hangs by my side in case I need a stabilizing force at any point.

I have been very blessed that my family has always been there for me – my wife, my sisters, my kids and my parents. I know that not everyone has that type of support system. At first, they didn't know everything that was going on with me because I didn't tell them. They knew I was having some problems, but it all came out when I had to get a pacemaker/defibrillator implanted in my chest. It's kinda hard to hide that. I told my out of town relatives that I was in the hospital, but it took months before I let them know that I almost died outside a racquetball court and several more times before and since. Now they know I've got this weird, rare heart disease that's causing me some serious problems. The cat came completely out of the bag when I went in for open heart surgery. There's not a whole lot you can say to brush that one off.

As I mentioned earlier, early on in my illness I thought I was being protective of my family - especially on the emotional side, because I wanted to steer them from being fearful. I figured that if they get fearful, then they probably would change the way they respond to me, and I didn't want them to. Each of them has specific things I depend on from them to help me get better. Having them shut down around me would disrupt my psyche, and change the way we interact. That proved to be inaccurate. As my older daughter pointed out to me multiple times, I need to communicate what's going on so they can worry less and be in a position to help me more.

Every family situation is unique as are the people who comprise it. Maybe you're reading this and don't have family that are close, or close by. Or maybe you don't have any family to rely on. If you do, keep in mind that your family members are only equipped to give you what they are capable of. You can't ask the super serious cousin to be a comedian. Or the one consumed by emotion to help you rationally think through your recovery. You've got to look at each one and ask what they can bring to the table and not be hesitant to tell them what you need from them. And, you can't be afraid to be upfront with what you need. If a family member isn't there, and you want them there, tell them. If they aren't helping your healing process the way you need, tell them.

I was advising a friend recently who has moved back home and her family doesn't understand the gravity of her situation or how she feels because she "looks" ok. They can't feel her aches and pains, her intense fatigue or the sick-to-your-stomach feeling she gets from all the meds she is taking. I told her to go on line and educate her family about her disease and the symptoms. It seems that the more rare the condition, the less people understand about how to help the patient cope with it. "Brand name" conditions like "cancer" or "stroke" are easier to see and understand, but no more serious or painful than many lesser known maladies.

If you are the family member, you have to realize the patient might not be comfortable asking you for help. In that case, turn it around and ask them. Ask your loved one's doctors and nurses, too: "What's my family member going to need when you send them home?" It might be a ride here or there, to cook some extra meals or just for someone to come by once or twice a week to chat. I've said it before. Assume that everyone who asks how they can help is genuine in their interest do something. So, as a patient, be specific with them. As the family member, offer up some ideas that might be helpful to the person trying to get better.

Now, not everyone has a strong family support system. If you need help, you might have to push beyond some of the issues of the past with those family members to say: "We've had some problems in the past, but this is what's happening and this would really help me now. I can't do this alone. Are you in a position to help me get through this?" If not, move on to whomever else you think you might be able to rely on. What's also important to remember is that your family is not your 24-hour caregiver, especially once you've recovered enough to be at home. They have their lives. They work, go to school, and they must be able to do those things. Understanding that as a patient is important. They have things they need and want to do, not just be Mr. Belvidere, the butler, at your beck and call all the time. Some family members (especially spouses) probably need the nudge to go ahead and do their thing, as it will also help them cope with your situation. One other thing to remember with your family: show your appreciation and give them credit and praise for all they do for you. At times, it seems to be just as hard being a loved one of a sick person as it is to be the patient. They go through the emotional ups and downs right along with you. Flash them a smile and give plenty of hugs for helping to keep you going.

My wife and kids do just that. They know me so well that they won't let me be a victim. Occasionally, if I'm looking a little dizzy or glazed over because my pills are knocking me out, Barb will knock on my chest and say, "Are you in there?" The inside jokes are important and show me we're all on the right page. The laughter is a coping mechanism for all of us. It's the "everything's going to be OK" signal.

When my dad went into the hospital and had all his complications, my sisters and I took on the caregiver role. It certainly is different when you are the one giving versus getting the care. You become: part motivational speaker, part dietician, part personal attendant, part waiter/waitress, part confidant, part counselor, part coordinator, part medical researcher, and part liaison with the rest of the world to keep them informed. There are several other elements to the job description, but you get the idea. The thing is to do what you can to support the person as they try to get better.

FIGHTING DISEASE FATIGUE

Of all the things you encounter on the road to getting better, disease fatigue might not be something you or any other patient ever thought about or is prepared to deal with. Of course, it goes without saying that the patient is tired of being sick. Aren't we all? Disease Fatigue is what happens to friends and family. The people who came to see you in the hospital may not check in with you very often when you get released and are back at home. That's when people tend to think: "OK, he/she must be better." In reality you might be out of the hospital, but not out of the woods. You're past the initial trouble and stabilized enough to go home, although still not well. In some cases, far from it. That's the case with sarcoidosis patients and hundreds of other ailments. Hospitals want you out asap these days. So do insurance companies. They lose money if you hang around complaining about the food and the cost of a $200 aspirin, or are aimlessly wandering around the hallways or playing cards with the other patients. Actually, most patients who can, want to heal at home anyway. My first question on every trip to the hospital was: "How soon can I leave?"

Here's an example of Disease Fatigue. Once you're out, people lose track of what's happening with you to some degree. Three months after I left the hospital after my first engagement there, I'm talking to the next door neighbor when he asks how I'm doing. In my usual way, I mentioned how I felt and how I'm still working to heal. He said, "I thought since you were out of the hospital that you were better. I just assumed everything was fine." Sometimes people make assumptions that you're healthy simply because you don't look sick on the outside. And it just never came up in our quick talks from one driveway to another as we came and went. I don't like going into detail about what's wrong with me except with very close friends or relatives, so it's rare for me to bring it up. People will assume you're healthy because they see you when you are up and around. They don't see you when you are down for the count. They don't know that the meds you're on make you sick to your stomach and that you have pain they can't see. Others don't know you wake up 10+ times a night, sometimes drenched in sweat. They see you walk, maybe slower, but under your own power, so they tend to assume the best and move on. When you've been sick for a while, you learn to mask your symptoms. You rub some proverbial dirt on it, walk it off (if you can) and deal with it.

This can be a difficult thing to handle for someone who's become accustomed to a certain level of attention and suddenly sees it drop off dramatically. If people can't "see" that you are sick, they will often assume that you are well. When they do see you, maybe they'll even tell you how good you look. Again, this is where the patient needs to set the tone for recovery by helping make sure the most important people in their life are informed. I have a group of college buddies who get a humorous update from me every few months. When I wanted to avoid disease fatigue with my old soccer teammates, I would "just show up" at a game. That brings me back into the loop. Work is easy. Just tell the office blabbermouth (who's always got her ears open for the latest gossip), and the entire company will know your status by lunch time.

Disease fatigue is another attack on the mental fitness part of getting better. It's not that people care less about you or your situation. In most cases, they probably just don't know what's happening. You know who to share information with, as well as who to limit what and how much you tell them. The important thing is to continue to set the tone and environment for your healing process. If that means sending email updates, creating your own personal website or reaching out to a few people by phone, don't be afraid to do it. Here's something I learned early on in my own 5-year home recovery process: Mental telepathy does not work and even my best friends can't read my mind. So don't be afraid to reach out to your friends. And, friends should ask if it is okay to share your situation with other friends in that circle. Getting an unexpected card in the mail can make a patient's day. I was home from the hospital and got a nice note from a long-time friend that I hadn't talked to in quite some time. I decided to pick up the phone and call to thank him. We talked for an hour and re-established our relationship. So, friends shouldn't hesitate to call, email, or send cards. After all, like the song says: "That's what friends are for."

SING-ALONG

Speaking of songs, they say that music soothes the savage beast. Well maybe it also works on bacteria, viruses, and other "beasts" inside your body that are trying to "unsoothe" you in any number of ways. Music can play a role in changing your mood and perhaps make you happier. Sometimes, you can draw inspiration or strength from a song that speaks to you in a certain way. If so, play it, sing it, read it. Put it on your phone, your iPod, your tablet and play it when you need it. You can even share it with others and use it to strike up a conversation. For me, there's a song that was written a couple decades ago called: *"This is it,"* by Kenny Loggins and Michael McDonald. This song has lyrics that speak to me because I see so much truth and connection to the words. I listen to this song and it's motivational. I can't sing it to you here – you'll have to wait for the audiobook version to hear my Queen Latifah meets Kermit the Frog voice. That aside, let me walk you through some of why the song has a strong meaning to me. Maybe you too can draw some strength from a song that speaks to you.

Kenny Loggins was singing to his dad. He encouraged him to "stand up and fight" and not wait for a sign or a miracle. In other words, things aren't going to get better on their own. You've got a big role to play in your own healing, and you can't be complacent about it. The theme of the song is that you can't just resign yourself that this is what you have and give up. You have an opportunity to get better in some aspect of your life.

This is the call to action. Figure out what you need and what you can do.

I used this song when I was sick, then one year after my open heart surgery, I went through this with my own dad. I introduced you to him earlier. When the doctor deemed him strong enough to undergo value replacement and triple bypass surgery, dad made the decision to do the surgery and set out with 3 goals in mind:

1. Dance at his grand daughter's wedding 6 months after the surgery.

2. Play golf again.

3. Be well enough to take care of his wife as he had done for the better part of 70 years.

He came through the nearly 6-hour surgery quite well, but then the complications started coming in high doses. One after another, they sapped the energy from his body and fight from his spirit. A 5-7 day stay turned into 22 days. Out for a week, then more complications and back in for another 10 days. Out for a week and back in for 2 more weeks including installation of a pacemaker.

My sisters and I stood vigil around his bedside. My job, as I saw it, was to help him fight through the mental part of the game that makes you want to give up. I'd been there, so I knew what it was like. I could see the struggle and pain on his face. I could feel the disappointment when the bad news kept coming day after day. Still, his surgeon said his "major" problems were fixed and if he could gut it out, he could recover.

Loggins goes on to tell his dad that there's nowhere to run and nowhere to hide – that his moment to decide is now. That's why the song was important for me. Once you're faced with a life threatening situation, you're there. Your back IS to the corner. Maybe the worst case scenario is there every day in the back or front of your mind. So, what are you going to do? You can't sit around and wait to get better. It might never happen. In my case, I was completely healthy, then, all of a sudden, out of nowhere, this awful disease appears. One day you think you're fine and the next day you're in the ICU. For my dad, he still had things he wanted to do and had been very healthy up to that point. Everyone who gets a serious illness is backed into a corner. You just have to make a decision about what are you are going to do and how you are going to go about getting out of it, or at least how you can make the best of it.

This hit home for me on the caregiver side as well. When my dad got sick, there were several weeks when he was in a lot of pain, ready to give up, call it a good life and shut down. I talked with him every day and every night. I knew what it was like to be in the bed and wondering if it was my time. He'd already been through so much pain and who could blame him for wanting to quit. But, although his mind was ready to shut down, his body wasn't. He was tolerating the treatments incredibly well, and there was still a good chance for recovery. If there was none, the conversations would have been different. But there was a chance. Every night as he tried to fall asleep we focused on one word. "Progress." That became our mantra. We'd review where he'd been, where he was, and where we were heading.

"This is it" has a self-confident tone to it. Nobody really believes they're going to have a major health problem. You always think: "I'm going to be around a long time." Illness is just not part of the song that you write for yourself. Then it happens and you're life changes. There's a line in the song about this. Things seem to be going along fine, the unexpected happens, and with "it," comes all the fear, anxiety and doubt – *"Now I'm not so sure."*

Then there's the discovery. The diagnosis comes back and your condition is confirmed. After the initial shock wears off – which can take weeks, you can go another direction. You first have to mentally say: Here's what I've got, now let me see how I can make the very best of this situation. Loggins sings to his dad about "…one good reason to try." I've got five good reasons – my family. That's plenty of motivation. When there's not good news, you might think the worst, but I've learned that even with a terminal disease, you can win small battles, and take it one day at a time. Often you wake up and are confronted with the first battle of the day – the mental one. It's takes a lot of effort to win each of these and they can sneak up on you at any time. Finding your own reason to try is critical.

The song ends with the family and friend part. The reassurance that no matter what you decide to do, I'll be by your side to support you. I told this to my dad many times, but added that if tomorrow showed "progress," there was a reason to do everything you can to survive, to get better, to win. If you're the patient, do it for yourself and the people who care about you. If you're the caregiver, assess the situation, talk to the doctors, talk to the patient and support them in the most positive way you can.

He finishes by saying that there comes a day in every life when you just have to make a choice of how it's going to play out – whatever "it" is. Maybe you're faced with adversity right now and maybe it's a life or death situation. What are you going to do? How are you going to face it? For me, as a parent, I wanted to project the right example. What's the example I'm going to set for my kids as I'm going through this? I want them to see their dad be strong through the process. Not whiny, not the "why me?" type stuff. Another line puts a lot of control back with the patient. "You make the choice of how it goes." To a large degree, it's what this book is about - all the choices you can make. If you do nothing, or if you just lay there and become a victim of your circumstance, that's a choice. I want my kids to say that their dad fought through whatever he had to fight through to get the most from every day. And, I want to share and celebrate the small wins with family and friends. Still, you may be completely incapacitated. I meet a lot of these folks when I volunteer at the hospital and visit the ICU and heart floors. Some are understandably and visibly upset…some to the point of giving up. I remember walking into the room of a young man, maybe 35 or 40 years old, just as the doctor was walking out. Apparently, he had just received the news that he had only 2 months to live. We talked for a long time. I was so impressed with how he was handling it and how he needed to get out of the hospital because he "had things to do." He told me that he was prepared. We prayed and he had tears in his eyes, but his voice was strong. It was the kind of strength that comes with a solid faith foundation. I can't imagine going through something like that with no belief system. His wife was in the room, showing strength and support. I asked if I could tell him a story about my time in the hospital. We shared a chuckle over some of the antics that I pulled off and I got the idea that he might be one of those guys who'd get up and write his own silly ideas on the treatment board in his room. His strength and resolve made an impression on me that I'll never forget. Every time I begin to think my situation is difficult, I meet someone who makes me ashamed of any "poor me" feelings that I might have.

Maybe you have something to say, show, do or share with someone who could use a compliment, encouragement or a smile. It might not seem appropriate, but maybe it's exactly what that person needs or wants at that moment. If you brighten their day in some way, you've helped them get better. Enough of those type "moments" can make for a better day.

The lyrics in "This is it" speak to me. They can help me to stay focused when I get distracted. Every time I hear it, I'm reminded that I have choices about how I'm going to get better in some aspect of my life.

What's your song? What song can provide you with a little extra motivation and drive to get better. "As Kenny Loggins says: "No one can tell what the future holds. You make the choice of how it goes. This is it." Absolutely right. So, let's get better.

WHO WANTS A MILKSHAKE?

One of the treatments I endured during my misdiagnosis period was something called IVIG. They use the acronym because Intravenous Immuno Globulin sounds really disgusting. This is a horrible mixture of antibodies taken from the plasma of something like 1,000 donors, which makes it absurdly expensive. Mine must have been mixed with Drano™ and vinegar because it made me ill – really ill. My first neurologist signed me up for this adventure at the oncology center, where all the patients with their various maladies sat in the semi-circular shaped Infusion Room to undergo 4-8 hour medicinal drip treatments. We all sat there looking at one another. It was like a séance for the sick. No one is happy to be there, and with good reason. It's a dreary, silent room where people of all ages and conditions kept to themselves while hooked up to IVs on the metal tree over their heads. People stared sullen faced at their individual TV monitors just passing their time watching some stupid show that they cared nothing about. After years of talking to rooms filled with excited salesmen and eager managers, I absolutely dreaded this place, not to mention the treatment itself which would take a physical and mental toll on anyone. These sessions involved sitting and looking around at nine other very sick people who all would rather be on jury duty than in this room.

On the day of my final treatment, I decided to change things up a bit. On the way to the center I stopped by the neighborhood Dairy Queen because I declared, to no one in particular, that

Friday would be Milkshake Day. I picked up 18 milkshakes and headed to treatment. I walked in carrying a tray reminiscent of something an old-time Vegas cigarette girl would have. By this time, the receptionist knew who I was, but still looked at me like I was nuts when I checked in. "Hi Kathy. Today is Milkshake Day!" I announced before offering her one of her own. She passed, but let me in with the goods. After dolling out a couple to the folks in the lobby, I headed back to the room of gloom and doom, put a big smile on my face, and broke the silence, "Hi, everybody. It's Milkshake Day!" I then walked to each of my fellow patients to give them a shake. I gave some to the nurses, too. They seemed a bit more energetic because of it. One elderly lady, who chose vanilla, asked me, "Is this new? I've never been here for Milkshake Day." Next was a young boy there for cancer treatment with his mother. She looked the way you'd expect a mom going through such an ordeal alongside her 9-year old would look. I offered the boy a shake, but he politely said no. "Are you kidding me?" I responded. "Take a sip if you like and share the rest with mom, who I know for a fact loves milkshakes." He laughed and they picked a strawberry shake to share. After distributing the goods, I grabbed a leftover chocolate and surprised the room by taking a seat and getting hooked up for treatment. People smiled and shouted a thank-you or two across the room. I yelled out something myself: "Nurse, we'd like to order lunch now!" Everyone laughed. I struck up a conversation with both the person on my left and right. Moods changed. Mission accomplished.

The goal was to break the somber mood in that room – to create a few smiles at least for that "moment." I admit that there was some selfish motivation in not wanting to sit there staring at 9 unhappy people for 4 hours. And, when you're going to spend half your day getting pumped full of some concoction that is going to make you feel worse instead of a lot better, you have to figure out how to make it bearable. Giggles and smiles elicited from the sucking sound of straws pulling in the last drops from the bottom of nearly empty cups told me it worked. Somehow, on that day, it was okay for everyone to make eye contact with their fellow patients and exchange smiles. That day was different. It worked for me and most of the folks in there that day. There were a couple people who didn't want to be there and didn't want a milkshake. That was fine by me. They were dealing with their own situation the best they knew how, and I had to remind myself that it's difficult for some people to cope with their circumstances and let down their guard. Bringing those people around might take some time. If that's you, find a way to lighten up a bit. Maybe grab a milkshake…and bring along a couple extra to share. It's guaranteed to make you feel better.

WE'RE OFF TO SEE THE WIZARD

Some people wouldn't get a joke if it knock-knocked them on their boney old head. Looking back, when we moved from New Jersey to Pennsylvania, I became the new kid in junior high. To try to fit in, I did what came naturally, and that was to "cut up" or fool around a little bit. It was just silly, stupid things, like yelling jokes across the room to my buddies. The French teacher, Mrs. Kasmala, did have to call my Mom in once (or was it twice) to talk about all of this cutting up that Tom, "Freck" and I were doing. As Ms. K related my unacceptable behaviors, she added some consolation to my Mom, "At the end of the day, they're disruptive, but at the same time, they're so damn much fun to have in class. They even make me laugh sometimes."

Mom kind of knew this already because at home, the silliness continued. Dad would still be dressed in his work finest for dinner and always help wash off the dishes afterward. For this, he'd wear an apron. That's when I'd sneak in behind him and tie the apron in knots. Dad would be grumbling and struggling trying to find his way out of his domesticated straight jacket. "Sorry, Dad, busy," I'd answer when he called to me to untie him. Mom liked to laugh and appreciated a good joke. Dad typically didn't get the humor – "That's not funny, @#$%&*%." I think he was chuckling on the inside and just went along with the game to appease me. The one time I can remember Dad actually all-out belly laughing was while he and I were channel surfing and landed on a Three Stooges movie. For some reason, on that day it just struck us both right in the funny bone. We both started laughing uncontrollably. You can't help but feel great after a good laugh. Sharing laughter is very powerful medicine indeed.

If you work at it, you can apply humor to most situations. In my world, that comes from having some great friends. They regularly email me stories, silly pics, stupid videos and other crazy stuff that keeps me laughing. My best friend and fellow knucklehead is Dave Lohr, a guy who I met in our Penn State fraternity days. To this day, we leave each other ridiculous voice mail messages and laugh like two guys on nitrous every time we talk. During the early stages of my illness, Dave had a serious brain abscess that required an operation to remove. He had to endure several months of IV drug treatments following his procedure. It's never that funny when someone saws off a piece of your skull. Fortunately, he came through and is just fine today. Another friend of ours, Joe was fighting bipolar issues. Ironically, Joe can be one of the funniest people to be around. Each of us had our own ailments to deal with. Dave sent us a greeting card with the characters from the Wizard of Oz on the front. Inside, he noted that this was us. He described our trio as the real life cast from The Wizard of Oz – He needed a brain, I needed a new heart and Joe needed some courage to face the day. My son Luke had a school dance around that time with the Wizard of Oz as the theme. Props were set up, so I took a picture of the life-sized cutouts of the Lion, Tin Man and Scarecrow, labeled it with our names and sent it off to the guys. Last time I was in the hospital, Dave sent me a Wizard of Oz paint by numbers gift as part of what was noted on the outside of my box as my "Recovery Kit." As I went through the contents and the accompanying "Instructions," that he wrote for me, my wife and I laughed until our sides ached.

It's the kind of humor you don't have to think about that is right in my wheelhouse. Most people might not get it, or think it was funny, but for the two of us it has an irony about it and the personal meaning attached enables us to laugh at our situations. During college, Dave and I would spend hours talking nonsense and writing stupid things on the fraternity house bulletin board to make light of posted items that were meant to be serious. Mostly, I think we entertained ourselves. After we graduated (no small miracle in itself), and before email, we sent, re-addressed and re-sent the same 9"x14" envelope through the mail to one another for over 10 years. I can't believe the post office would even deliver the thing. I'm happy to say the silliness continues to this day. I kid him about spending too much time scanning the internet to find stupid pictures and videos of funny things in the moment. Sometimes, he doctors up the pictures by putting my face or that of our friends into the scene for an added kick. So my recommendation is this: If you're a patient, find someone who can make you laugh. If you're a caregiver, lighten the mood with a funny story from the past or a joke you run across. Goofy? Yes. Therapeutic? Absolutely. No matter where I'm at or what the situation is, I look for an opportunity laugh or smile with someone. And, you can usually get a smile out of someone just by being nice to them. Smiles are contagious. They open the door to laughs. Laughing makes you feel better - and that completes the circle.

I talk with Dave on the phone every other week or so and there probably aren't 3 days that go by without receiving a ridiculous email. Our buds: Murph, George and Paul chime in regularly as well. They probably have no clue how much I appreciate them all and value their friendship. Maybe you know someone (or are someone) who needs a laugh. If laughter is the best medicine, then my friends are some of my best physical therapists and I don't know what I'd do without them. They've helped me through some very difficult times without even realizing it. Thanks guys.

IT DOESN'T COST
ANYTHING TO BE NICE

Another side of healing came from a great guy I grew up with named Jimmy Rallis who worked taking payments at a parking lot in our small town. Jimmy had a smile on his face for each person he met and just a great way with people. I came by to say hello one day and after witnessing one of his moment-making interactions, I asked him about his good-natured demeanor. His reply was simple – "it doesn't cost anything to be nice to people." Jimmy died of a brain aneurysm way before his time. I've always tried to keep his approach in mind as I go through each day as my personal tribute to him. I think about him a lot and he was right. It doesn't cost anything to be nice to our friends, family, strangers, nurses, doctors…even our phlebotomists. Open a door for someone, hold the elevator instead of rushing to close the door, toss a compliment their way, or just say "good morning." And smile more. It's often the simple things that make the difference. Each of these situations can make you feel good…and they don't cost anything.

YOU CAN TAKE IT WITH YOU

When you've got that "be nice" spirit going for you, it travels with you everywhere. In the hospital, I wanted to keep things as light as possible with the nurses, food providers and anyone else who could help me to focus elsewhere and feel better. Again, I might have to set the tone to let them know it's OK to be a little playful or bust my chops. In the process, it's giving those employees a chance to have fun with their job. If that mindset goes with them into the next room and it becomes OK for them to open up and relax, then they become better at helping people get better. It's one of those "I'm in a great mood" kind of things. Whether you just feel poorly or are really sick, and even though it is difficult sometimes, take some steps to remain in a good frame of mind. This strategy might just serve you well in moving past the minor aggravations that illness brings with it every day.

Now, of course, there are times when you don't feel funny. Maybe you just feel completely fatigued or really ill, or maybe in some level of pain or discomfort. Finding ways to fight through these periods isn't easy, but I've found it to be essential. It would be easy to throw a pity party. After all, if you are a patient reading this, you are certainly not where you want to be. I'm sure your condition reminds you of this. My disease reminds me every time I walk up a flight of stairs, attempt physical activity or when I get up from a chair too quickly. I've even become accustomed to feeling sick to my stomach from sun up to sun down on certain days. To weather these storms,

I can always write a short note to my friends describing a funny situation and they'll reply with their own brand of humor. It simply lightens the load.

My job for the last 25 years has been working with groups of business owners, managers and front-line employees to help them adopt new behaviors so they can improve at their job. After a short time in a hospital bed, I wanted to figure out how I could influence the behaviors of the people walking into my room. That goes for caregivers, relatives and friends. I don't want anyone in a panic or wearing "that face" – you know the gloomy one I'm talking about – the "oh my God you look terrible" face when they come in to see you. I had this conversation with one of my work friends, Elizabeth. She has adopted this theme whenever she sees me by putting on a big smile and telling me: "Hey Mark, you don't look like hell today."

Influencing behavior in a positive way is especially important for caregivers and for everyone who works in a hospital or doctor's office. I watched what the nurses have to deal with throughout every day. What a tough job it must be to work and build relationships with a group of sick people who come and go, and some that never leave. How do they deal with that reality of their job every day? Does it take away some of the human element of being a care provider? Do they take it home with them at night? These questions fascinated me, so I continually thought about how they were dealing with a wide range of patients and potential outcomes. I reached the conclusion that the experiences they have with their patients are what can make or break the day. Again, I asked myself, how can I help them to help me (and my fellow patients) to heal. Since I could only go so far in controlling my physical outcome, I decided to keep things light and get them to smile with me as much as possible. That would help the mental part of the game that puts a patient in the healing mindset. It can help family and visitors as well.

SHENANIGANS

Just about the first thing you notice while stuck in a hospital bed (well, perhaps after the wide variety of wires and tubes now attached to you like ropes holding a boat at dock) is the prominently placed dry erase "Treatment Board" on the wall of your room. The board tells everyone who the doc on call and current nurses are, as well as some other details of meds and special treatments for the day. I mentioned earlier that I used this to cue up my "massage" with Nurse Sarah. When I saw that whiteboard, my inner child immediately thought: "This is just too good to pass up." So, with no medical training – and I've never played a doctor on TV, either – I started to write my own ridiculous treatments on the board. One of my "instructions" stumped a new nurse. She walked in and introduced herself, "Hi, I'm Mary." I looked at her very matter-of-factly and said, "Hi, Mary. Are you here to take my ear wax samples?" She looked stunned and replied, "No one told me anything about that." I promptly directed her attention to the dry erase Treatment Board where it was written quite clearly: "Take ear wax samples." Clearly perplexed, she read the board with a stupefied look that said she didn't quite know what to do next. I, of course, decided to continue the ruse showing her what my mom refers to as "my nice Ukrainian ears" (whatever that means). As we started to discuss the virtues and possible purposes of ear wax evaluation, another nurse who knew me pretty well by then, walked into the room. Mary asked, "Do you know anything about the ear wax samples?" The other nurse replied, "What?" Then she glanced at the board and looked over to see me smiling (appropriately) ear to ear. "You're not listening to him, are you? He wrote that himself." We all had a good laugh. And now she was in a better frame of mind to be both clinical and to some degree, more comical. Mission accomplished.

Humor during difficult times is the opposite of what most people think about when things go south. It's a reaction and a response we aren't supposed to have when things get bad. It's not that I'm discounting the seriousness of your situation or mine, I'm just trying my best not to succumb to it. It's my defense mechanism for fighting anxiety and/or depression. I also figure that if I'm going out, I'm going out with a smile on my face. When someone has to give my eulogy, I want them to have some good material. The dim mood of a hospital bed or bed at home might not seem like the best place to be cutting up or just flat out being silly, but that's exactly why it is the perfect place to do it. That's why I chose to do it and it might just help you loosen up and cope with your situation. One thing for sure is that it will give a few people more than their share of chuckles. It also gave me something other than my condition, to talk about with family and visitors. I needed the diversion, so I tried to entertain myself as best I could during my stints in the hospital, and even appointed myself the unofficial Floor Social Chairman. Every morning after my 5am wake-up call from the bloodsuckers, I'd write up and post a bogus "TODAY'S ACTIVITIES" sheet outside my room for all to see. After a couple days, the nurses would gather around my door to see what was planned for the day. Keep in mind that most patients on the Heart Floor, myself included, had very limited mobility.

On the next pages are some of the daily activity sheets I posted around the floor during my stay. Intentionally silly for sure and deliberately done to get a reaction. I laughed while I wrote them and took pleasure when I shared them with another patient or heard people talking or snickering about my latest creation in the hallway. It's the simple fun of having people stand outside the door and enjoy the fact that someone can take their situation and make the best of it – even in the ICU or heart recovery wing of a hospital. Maybe it gives that person, especially if it's a caregiver, a smile and changes the way they interact when they walk in your room. And, maybe they can have a funny story to tell when they go home at night.

TODAY'S ACTIVITIES, MONDAY, MARCH 1

4 a.m. to 6 a.m.: Rock, Paper, Scissors Day w/the lab girls (you win, no shots).

6 a.m. to 8 a.m.: Monthly "off-the-diet" breakfast (cheese-covered eggs, bacon, sausage, biscuits and gravy, choice of cream-filled chocolate donuts or cherry cheese Danish, juice or Diet Coke).

9 a.m.: Water aerobics with Nurse Mary (Bring your bed pan)

11 a.m.: Morning lecture: Sleep deprivation and its impact on the patient-nurse relationship

Noon: Lunch on your own

2 p.m.: Patient Hula Hoop contest.

4 p.m.: Afternoon lecture: The Art of ripping off adhesive bandages from all parts of the body.

6 p.m. to 8 p.m.: Progressive Dinner (We'll start with drinks and appetizers in Room 8623).

8 p.m. to 2 a.m.: Poker Night (Phlebotomists welcome).

TODAY'S ACTIVITIES, TUESDAY, MARCH 2

4 a.m.: Labwork (canceled).

9 a.m.: Breakfast cocktail mixer (bring your meds).

11 a.m.: Tango lessons with Nurse Lisa.

Noon: Lunch 'n Learn: Existentialism

2 p.m.: Wheelchair Races vs. 6th Floor (We've never lost to the 6th floor, so get psyched people).

4 p.m.: Nurse Commando's hospital gown fashion show.

6 p.m.: Pot Luck Dinner (bring a dish).

8 p.m.: Bingo!

LET ME ENTERTAIN ME

Some people probably thought I was nuts, but the goal was never to win people over. My intention for these activity sheets and stuff like the contest to make the best hospital glove chicken (which I won, thank you very much. Never mind that I was the only participant) was twofold: 1) To take my attention away from thinking about dying – which was a distinct possibility at the time, and 2) to make it easier for people to walk into my room. It was an opportunity to lessen the tension between caregiver or visitor and patient, and create a less anxiety-filled interaction. Imagine the difference when someone walks into your room already smiling and starts the conversation lightheartedly instead of with a heavy heart. For me, it made all the difference in the world. I didn't feel like I was dying. I felt like I was getting better.

Another benefit came on the family side. When my kids came by and they read the stuff on my door before walking into my room, I had them primed for a good visit. It eased their minds a bit because they're thinking: "Dad's being Dad." Luke and Nicholas found the stuff hysterical, Elise and Olivia would kind of roll their eyes the way only daughters can when they think their father is being a goof. My wife pretty much just ignored my antics - which came from decades of practice.

On the next page, is one more Daily Activity posting. It contains several activities that are my personal favorites:

SUNDAY'S ACTIVITIES

5 a.m.: *Good Morning wake-up call: Meet your phlebotomists.*

6:30 a.m.: *Disney character breakfast*

8 a.m.: *Decorate your bed for the monthly bed pan parade.*

9 a.m.: *Parade.*

10:30 a.m.: *Waterless shower tips w/Nurse Sara.*

Noon: *Pie-eating contest and weenie roast (1st floor cafeteria).*

2 p.m.: *Group Presentation: How to operate the damn bed (large conference room).*

3 p.m.: *Kickboxing w/PCTs Sam and Brandy.*

4 p.m.: *Morale Booster: Watch CNN for 20 minutes and feel how lucky we are to be in here.*

6 p.m.: *Med Mixer: You do mine, I do yours.*

8 p.m.: *Who can make the best chicken out of a blown up glove contest.*

10 p.m.: *We all bust out of here and go to Quigley's for some real shots.*

FLIP THE SWITCH

Ok, I understand that some of you reading this are probably thinking that I should have been moved from the Heart Wing to the Psychiatric Ward. Not a bad idea. Think of the fun you could have in there! Problem with that is I wanted to go home and they might never have let me out.

When visitors venture out of the patients room, they might find themselves in another depressing place. Waiting rooms, for example, are no fun either. The TVs are showing the days bad news or some absurd soap opera – never ESPN or reruns of Seinfeld. If you don't recreate the environment for yourself, the environment will dictate a response for you. I don't like the thought of that. For me it's all about feeling better as a person, as well as being healed physically. After all, it took me 4 years to begin to heal physically to the point where I felt somewhat "good" again. And, I surmised that if the people around me aren't feeding me positive stimulus, I'm not going to heal as quickly. At least, this is what I think to be true; if you have to eat hospital food, feed yourself some positive energy along with it. It's too easy to get weighed down by the bad stuff. You've already got enough issues to deal with without piling negativity on the heap of dirty laundry. It reminds me of one trip to the cardiologist's office, a regular stop on my journey to getting better. There was a 70-something gentleman in a wheelchair just smiling and saying hello to everyone who'd make eye contact with him. You could tell he was a real character. A nurse asked him how he was doing and, without missing a beat, he says: "well, I had a 10-mile run this morning, so I'm a little sore." (He could barely get out of his wheelchair). I'm laughing along with him and admiring his spirit. Before he came in the room, everyone else in the waiting room was so stoic with no facial expressions, no conversation and certainly no happiness. He was so loud that he changed the mood of the office. Others might have grumbled, but I thought it was great. I said to myself: "Man, if I can make it through the next 15 years, that could be me!"

That guy flipped the energy switch on during my heart clinic visit, which is something I always tried to do in the hospital, especially with the staff. They made my stay much more bearable. If I hadn't lit the fuse, we would have never had fireworks. I like fireworks. As you might have guessed, I also like to upset the apple cart a little bit. I want to catch people off guard. The fun thing is anyone can do it in their own way. After surgery, I was ordered to get up and walk around the floor as much as possible. Here's the sign I put on my door:

If I'm not here, it is likely that I have made a break for it and am looking for a way out of here. (I usually don't make it too far, so come on in and sit down).
- Mark

BREAKING OUT/STICKING TOGETHER

Escaping from the Hospital, at least our plot to do so, turned out to be a great ice breaker for meeting some of my fellow floor mates. I had mentioned it on one of the daily activity sheets posted on the floor.

*10 p.m.: **We all bust out of here and go to Quigley's for some real shots.***

Then, during one of my first nighttime shuffles –(the act of walking without lifting your feet) – down the hall, I stopped by the room of a guy named Bob. We'd talked a little before, mainly because I'd always be on the lookout for other people to engage during my shuffles. So, Bob is sitting there with his wife when I pass by. He asks me how things are going. I say, "I'm busting out of here tonight to get a beer. Are you with me?" Bob, almost on cue, whispers, that he's got the tunnel half dug out already, but needed a plan for the dirt. I decided I can take care of the dirt by employing the same trick they used in the classic movie "The Shawshank Redemption." I'd put the soil in my pajama pockets and inconspicuously spread it out in the hallway. We carried on the ruse a bit longer and chuckled about it quite a bit.

The same night, I shuffled down the hall and met another gentleman named Steve who had just had a quadruple bypass.

I filled him in on the escape plan to break out and go hit Quigley's for a beer: "The guy two doors down is digging the tunnel, I'm spreading dirt in the hall so they won't notice." Steve says he'll bring "the wallet" – then pointed to his brother-in-law who was visiting at the time – to bankroll our night out. Continuing to play along, I told the brother-in-law, that it was good he had some money because I had left my wallet in my other smock. The conversation progressed to other things and went on for several more minutes. His wife mentioned later how much she appreciated the ridiculous banter. Spouses, relatives and friends go through an illness right along with the patient to some degree. I guess at that moment, it helped her feel better too.

Something we had in common was that we all had "serious" conditions. I tried to lighten the mood by sharing a trick that I played on the nurses or showing them the award-winning chicken I decorated from a blown up hospital glove. It's hard not to smile when the person talking to you just presented you with a latex chicken. And, here's the thing – if their family was in the room looking all worried and serious, it would lighten them up as well. We'd get into a conversation and actually start laughing about something...anything. Next day when I'd be shuffling by they'd invite me in with a smile and the conversation would move from our maladies to lighter fare. We'd chat about how fashionable our gowns were, the dumb show on the TV, my ridiculous bedroom slippers, or the decision whether to order the trout almondine with capers or the bacon-wrapped filet mignon for dinner – neither of which were a possibility, of course. Conversations would lighten up and by the time it was time to move on, <u>everyone</u> in the room was feeling better. My patient friend, Bob, was two doors down and recovering from quadruple bypass surgery. After a couple conversations, whenever he saw me walking by, he'd initiate the conversation and make me laugh. He got discharged several days before me and I missed him. I wish that I would have grabbed his email.

(Bob, if you read this, call me). I saw firsthand how letting the air out of the "let's be serious" balloon helped me to forget about my problems – at least for a while – and just maybe it did the same for my patient friends and their families. Figure out how you can try this with your friends and family. And for all you visitors, try this with the patient you're going to see and watch what happens.

Like everything else in this book (and in life), there's no guarantee that this will work in every situation, or with every patient. Many of my friends know I'm sick and think maybe the meds are getting to me as well. Maybe they are right on both counts. I was lucky to be alive when I entered the hospital and every day I am grateful to God for the strength to battle this disease and for the gift of another day. Every so often something happens and that slice of medical reality confronts me, but I am now mentally prepared to deal with it. Some might say I don't want to face the reality of my situation. Maybe that's true, but I'm going to stick to my strategy nonetheless. The ideas and antics in "Getting Better" are coping mechanisms that might just give you strength to face your illness (or your loved ones) at some level. I'm not suggesting that you do what I did and am doing. I learned what worked for me through a lot of trial and error. I'm still learning today…and still applying some new ideas each day…and if God thinks it might be fun to see how I'll respond to whatever he tosses my way tomorrow, then I'll thank Him for the extra 24 hours and set out to make Him proud.

Here's another thing about lightening up a bit: You'll know within your first few attempts how the other person will respond. For me, playing around with my family and friends and catching them off guard is another step in the recovery process. If it doesn't work, you've lost nothing, but if it works, you've just made life much more pleasant for yourself and those around you and that's not such a bad thing.

BONDING

Some important bonds are formed in the hospital and doctor's office. Patients with patients, staff with patients, sometimes families with families, dogs with cats, etc. For humans, it comes out of the common circumstances of being on the same boat. We might be in different cabins, but we're all on the same boat – the SS Recovery. You never know when the opportunity to bond will present itself and you'll never know who you might meet. One day shuffling along, I spotted an older gent in his room who looked familiar. I knocked on the door and said, "I think I know you." I didn't know him personally, but it was a man named Don who I recognized as an usher at our church. We'd been acknowledging one another via head nod and smile on Sundays for years. However, he didn't know my name and the only reason I knew his was the name tag he wore with the title "Usher" underneath. Don needed bypass surgery and had a slew of complications. We chatted and became fast friends. How fast? Two days after formally meeting we're talking when a nurse walks in with his meds. Don turns to the nurse and he says, "Come back later, can't you see I'm talking to my buddy?" After a couple of conversations, I'm his buddy! Don was an interesting guy with some fascinating stories about his life growing up in our little town. Our maladies weren't a topic of discussion usually, just the reason we connected. Shortly after I left the hospital, I learned that Don had passed away. It was very sad news for me to hear. I had intended on several occasions to go see him after we both were released, but I never made it over in time. To this day, I regret that I didn't get to see him again and think about him often. From now on, when I want to see a friend, I'm going right away. Maybe you have someone who is ill that you'd like to see. Don't wait until it's too late. Go…and bring some cookies and a funny movie.

620 HAD A BOWEL MOVEMENT

When you stop for a second to look around, you see that life is both fragile and funny. It might not seem obvious, especially as you're fighting illness in the hospital, but the little things you see and hear make you realize it's OK to look for reasons to laugh and smile. I'm sitting in bed one early morning during my hospital stay and overheard two nurses strike up a "business" conversation in the hall. "Hey, Mary, 620 had a bowel movement!" one said. "Oh, that's great … Did you document it?" the other excitedly responded. You'd never hear that conversation anywhere else. I'm just sitting in bed belly laughing over this silly conversation I just heard about some guy a few doors down who finally pooped. And, here's these two nurses talking about it like the guy won a special recognition award from the Chamber of Commerce. And to them, this was a perfectly normal conversation. I couldn't keep myself from laughing which was rather painful considering my condition. It was just so ludicrous. The observational stuff – the normally abnormal and stupid things that people say and do around us – is just so easy to laugh at. I've always gotten a kick out of storytelling, especially when you can poke fun at yourself in the process. Before I got sick, I'd take the humor in everyday life and churn it up a little bit for the sake of a laugh. Like telling the kids about how one time Dad left for work with one brown shoe and one black shoe, which can happen when you're not totally with it at 5 a.m., except that one had laces and the other was a slip on. Silly stuff like that. The kids, who like to blame the meds for some of my occasional loopiness, also gave me a courtesy laugh after my story about a call to the insurance company when I mistakenly asked whether I had reached "Northwestern _Musical_." The polite lady on the other end of the call said, no, I had called Northwestern _Mutual_. I responded the only way I could think, "Perfect, would you connect me to the trombone department please?"

You might not "feel" like you are funny, but that doesn't mean you can't be happy. Don't get me wrong. I'm not happy with my circumstances – far from it. However, here I am and I'm happy for that. I find that you sometimes have to search hard to find <u>something</u> positive or to discover a way to make the best of the situation you're in. I think I've tried over 100 different things in the last few years. Maybe "the search" itself can help with coping, healing or even happiness. After all who wants to live the rest of their life unhappy?

Here's another tip: Maybe you're saying to yourself: "that's just not me." Or "I'd never do that." That's OK. Just being pleasant works. One contagious condition you can catch in a hospital – or anywhere is Smiling Syndrome. Catch a smile and give it to someone. Or return a smile to someone whose infectious grin comes your way. If you don't think you are funny, find someone who is – a friend or relative who always has a good story, a joke to tell or is just one of those people who can make you laugh with normal conversation. Don't be afraid to let them know that you've always appreciated their ability to make you smile. Ask them to bring some of their sunshine into your day - if not in person, then by phone or email. Try this with the next person that you come across. As soon as they walk in the room, greet them with a smile and say something along the lines of: "Hi, I was hoping you'd come by. How are you?"

BEING SICK ISN'T SUPPOSED TO BE FUNNY

Being sick isn't funny. It's all the other goofy stuff that happens around you when you are sick that can be. It's hard to see humor in situations when you're hurting, scared, and really ill. I found that I had to train myself to look for it. To seize any opportunity to smile, laugh or just be happy in the moment. It was more about self-preservation than trying to be a comedian. I didn't want to fall into the abyss of discouragement and depression. They told me the meds I'm on could bring on these emotions and I didn't want any part of that. It's hard enough when there are thoughts going through your head that there's a good chance you won't make it through the ordeal you are facing. I know firsthand how this felt when the options were laid out in front of me and none of them were good. The point is that it is all too easy to fall into the trap of "I'm not supposed to be happy because I am sick." Pulling out of that mindset takes regular, sometimes continuous practice, and sometimes requires a little help from your friends.

TIPS FOR SMILING MORE

There are a couple of important pieces to remember in all this talk about fun and laughter:

1. Start with a smile and encourage others to do the same, or just find ways to be generally nice to people. Let them see that the real you is still in there.

2. It's OK to lighten the mood, in or out of the hospital and especially at home, by bringing some humor into the picture. Try it and see what happens. See how you feel at that moment.

3. If you don't make it known that people can have fun with you, then the nurses will be more serious, the docs will be more uptight and your loved ones will sit and stare at you with that look of fear or pity on their face. And who needs that?

4. You need support, so set the tone and let people know it's just fine to have fun with you despite your situation.

5. Ask your family or friends to send or bring you a book, magazine, video, cartoon, YouTube link or anything to make you smile, then share what strikes your funny bone with them. Read it back to them or watch it together. It may be even more funny the second time when you are sharing it with someone.

6. Seek out people who can make you smile and let them know they are helping you to heal just by being who they are. They'll appreciate it and you'll feel better as a result.

PRAYING FOR THE BEST

Oh no, here comes the part where he tries to convert us!

Sorry to disappoint you, but I'm not going to give a sermon, thump a Bible or beg for money like some of those late night evangelistic fundraisers with the big hair and $4,000 suits. And would someone tell these people that "God" is not pronounced with 2 syllables. I'm sure we'd all like to be cured by a good slap in the forehead with a healer's palm, convulse a few times and fall backwards to be caught by 2 ex-bouncers from the C&W bar down the road. But, for most of us, it doesn't work that way. My purpose is only to tell you about my experience – where I was and where I am with this very complicated thing we call our Faith. And if some of it makes sense to you, great. Maybe you can draw strength from connecting with your higher source.

People have been praying for me since I was a little kid. Given the exuberance of my youth, I probably needed more prayers than most. I'm quite sure my Mom would look at me in church while I was growing up, shake her head, and start praying … really hard. Through my current healing process I realized that I didn't ever really pray for myself. I prayed for other people – the wife and kids, my parents, aunts, uncles, other people who were sick, everyone else, just never for myself. Maybe I was too egotistical to believe that I needed prayers, who knows? Even if you're not particularly religious or haven't been to church in years, I believe prayer can help. I believe that now more than ever. I've had several doctors tell me that they have seen recoveries that have no basis in science. Perhaps you or a loved one are in that boat. Maybe doctors should start prescribing this right along with the meds they pump into our bodies. Know someone who needs a prayer? Clasp your hands together and say a few words to the Almighty. Maybe it will help you too. It certainly can't hurt. Do you think God listens even more carefully when an atheist starts to pray? I visualize God turning his head, looking right at the nonbeliever with a surprised look on his face and saying (with a south Chicago accent): "You talkin' to me?"

Religion has always been a part of my family's life. I was raised Roman Catholic, went to church on Sundays, endured elementary school with the nuns back when they could beat you with a ruler whether you deserved it or not - without fear of repercussions. I made my First Communion, Confirmation, and attended religious education classes all through high school. The family went to church every Sunday and I went along for the ride. The faith of Mark (me, not the apostle) was more going through the motions because it was the right thing to do, not necessarily because I had the strong inner faith that some others had. That's not to say I didn't believe in God. I did and I still do. It's just that things are different now.

After high school and college, I continued to go to church weekly and I prayed occasionally. As life changed, I prayed more. When the kids started arriving and as they were growing up, my faith grew stronger. I had no choice. By the time Barbara and I had four children waking up in our house in the morning and showing up late at night, we were doing a lot of praying.

As your kids are growing, a lot of stuff is happening and you find yourself praying for their health, safety, protection from evil, and that they make good decisions and walk the right path. The majority of my prayerful times came at the dinner table saying grace and in moments of reflection at church, and of course, by the kid's bedsides when putting them to sleep.

Over the years, my wife has gone from being devout to being very devout. She's stepped up her game big time, but never really pushed me. Here's the thing. When I got sick, I knew that she and the kids were praying for me along with a ton of our friends, and even people that I didn't know at church. Somehow, that was comforting. It was the first time that I really appreciated that people were praying for me or began to understand what that meant.

Being a weekend Christian, I had my doubts that prayer was actually working during the week. So many people say "I'll be praying for you," but I took it with a grain of salt (or Mrs. Dash™ as I'm not allowed to have salt), because I never recognized the power of prayer in my own personal life growing up. That's not to say I didn't "experience" the power of prayer. I just didn't recognize it. You have to actually look for something if you want to find it. When I look back, I see that God's been answering my prayers for my entire life. It was easier to take things for granted that they just happened rather than give the glory to God when they did. When people would say they were praying for me, I just didn't know if they really were or if it was just something to say given the situation. I didn't know if it made any difference. It wasn't until I crashed and thought there was a good chance I was dying that the power of prayer truly revealed itself to me. I think some of my fellow patients might relate to this.

BACK TO THE O.R.

One afternoon while in the hospital, a nurse rushed into the room and announced they were taking me to the OR for a heart biopsy procedure *right now* that involved scraping a few samples from the inside of my heart to try to figure out what was wrong. Apparently, my team of cardiologists were discussing my case and consulting with a specialist who had the skills to perform a certain delicate biopsy in some areas of the heart which should not be messed with. It caught Barbara and I off guard, to the point that she was visibly shaken by the idea of this spontaneous procedure. So, the nurse says I have to sign this "it's not their fault if I die" document, which I politely declined until after I talked to a doctor to find out why this was so urgent. They said I could do that downstairs and started to wheel me out anyway. Just then, at that very moment, I met Father Pat for the very first time. He was the hospital Chaplain making his rounds and happened to be at my door at that exact moment in time. Of the 300+ beds in this huge facility, he shows up right there right then…Divine intervention? Maybe. We stopped for a moment and he asked if I'd like to receive the sacrament of the Anointing of the Sick. I said yes. He blessed me and said a quick prayer. It gave me peace. Barbara as well. After that, I had no doubt that God would take care of me. There was no question in my mind that the procedure would go perfectly and I'd be fine. It didn't hit me until later, but that level of comfort and confidence is what Faith is all about.

Father Pat told me later that I had a smile on my face as they wheeled me out for that surgery. "Most people see me and think the Grim Reaper is right behind me," he quipped to me. My smile was, in part, because of seeing him, but also because he brought with him, the faith and confidence that God was going to take care of me. By that point, there just wasn't any fear. A big part of that came from prayers said for me, with me and by me. Still not sure if prayer is for you? Maybe you should pray on it.

THE PROS FROM DOVER

I recall a M.A.S.H. episode where Hawkeye and Trapper go to Seoul to work on a General and refer to themselves as the "Pros from Dover." The cardiologist, who entered through a series of opening doors like something out of a Get Smart episode (minus the shoe phone), was Dr. Maria Rosa Costanzo. This was our first encounter. She told me what was going on and said she'd met with the other cardiologists and this was the next course of action. They agreed that she should perform this procedure and she asked if there was an OR and team available. Just by luck (or was it more than luck?), there was, so we were a "Go" right then – thus the sudden nature of the situation. She even got a chuckle in the operating room when I turned the tables on her and asked if she got plenty of sleep the night before. Dr. Costanzo knows cardiac sarcoidosis and I am blessed to have her now coordinating my care with all the other physicians involved. Over the last couple years, we've developed a special rapport that enables her to be very straightforward with me and enables me to be myself. She gives me confidence that, though it is by no means easy, we are on the right path. I can feel that she cares deeply and truly wants to help me get better. That's very comforting for a patient. And I'm on a first name basis with her staff Mary and Kim, who also know me as a person, not just a faceless patient or case.

I went into this surgery completely relaxed and fully expecting to come out of it with no complications. There was no fear. Faith and prayer can do that. On the table in the OR surrounded by doctors and nurses, one of them asked how I was doing. "I'm great. More importantly, how are you all doing?" I quipped in response. Everyone chuckled. That was my way of lightening the mood to get in the right frame of mind for an unpleasant procedure that started with a giant nail-sized needle being jabbed in my jugular vein. By the way, thank goodness for the other pros from Dover, the anesthesiologists. They're sneaky fellows who you mostly see upside down as they look down on you from head to toe for about 10 seconds. Nine. Eight. Seven. Six. Five. Four. Thr......... They just kind of sneak in and knock you out. Next thing you know, you're waking up to someone saying, "You're all done." In all the procedures that I've had, I don't remember the names of any of the anesthesiologists (sorry guys), so I just call them all Dr. Knockout. Works for me. They put you to sleep, then have to wake you up...kind of like your mom did when you were in elementary school.

FAITH HEALERS

After that procedure, things changed. I could almost feel the prayers coming in my room and giving me strength to deal with whatever would come next (and there was a lot to come next that I had no clue was coming). It moved me to know the congregation at our church prayed for me during Sunday Mass. I got a visit from Deacon Joe from our church as he was making his rounds at the hospital. We've since become good friends and he even joined me on my exercise walks a few times a month when the weather was warm. He says he prays for me every morning. I have lots of people telling me this. Wow. Just knowing so many people were asking God to help me through this ordeal proved to be very comforting. Maybe it's why I'm still here. One thing I know: It worked for me and maybe it can work for you.

I volunteer at the hospital now bringing Communion to patients in the ICU and heart wing. It's amazing to me how many people want me to pray with and for them. Many were like me and never really prayed for themselves before. I think it helps me with my ongoing effort to get better as well. Sometimes they are in good spirits and sometimes in dire shape. Sometimes we laugh and smile as we talk about their situation and sometimes there are tears. Most times there is appreciation that someone cares enough to listen and pray for them and their family. Sometimes the nurses join in. Maybe that's appropriate as these people are Saints in my book.

Father Pat came back a few days after the surgery. He came by to pray with me, something I was now getting used to, and to give me a rosary. It was bright green macramé, nothing all too fancy, but made by a soldier friend of his. I've had rosaries in the past, just never carried or even used them. I tied it to my hospital bed. It truly is one of those things you can draw a lot of strength from just by looking at it and knowing it is there. Unlike the charlatans on TV who we talked about earlier, the rosary is a real faith healer. So I decided to share it.

A few doors down was my buddy, Don, the usher at our church. During one of my shuffling trips I stopped in to visit him. He was nervous about his upcoming procedure, so I asked whether he'd like to pray together. (I figured it brought me a lot of comfort and maybe it could for him). He said yes, so we said a few prayers. Later, I went back to give him the rosary I had received from Father Pat as I thought it might bring him some comfort.

Father Pat visited me again soon after, and I told him about giving the rosary to Don, who was getting ready for a serious surgery of his own. Father Pat said he hoped I would do something like that, sharing it with someone else who could benefit or use it. It's not that I didn't need it; Lord knows I did…it's just that Don needed it too. He and I then went to Don's room and we all prayed together. Father Pat and I became friends and before he moved on to another assignment, I made it a point to give him a call when I was at the hospital just to say hello.

A couple weeks after I got out of the hospital, I ran into Don's wife in church, she made it a point to tell me Don was also out of the hospital and now had that rosary tied to his bed at home. His wife told me that he loved it and kept it close throughout his ordeal even after being discharged. I thought that was pretty neat. You do these little things that don't appear to mean too much at the time. You think they might help, but you're not in the habit of doing them. Then you see they have an impact. Before getting ill, I rarely prayed with anyone unless they asked me to. I never said, "Do you want to pray on this?" to people. I started to see the power of an active commitment to faith. Today, I feel different, more comfortable, more confident. I've had the opportunity to pray with hundreds of people when volunteering at the hospital and I'm amazed at how receptive people are even if they say that they are not very religious. As I mentioned earlier, Don passed away shortly after being discharged. When I attended his viewing and funeral, I was surprised to see the green rosary positioned in Don's hands as he lay in the casket. That vision chokes me up still to this day.

JUST SAY IT

Not long after my surgery, I found myself back at my cardiologist's office after waking up drenched in sweat with a high temperature and crazy heart rate. It was tied to some changes with my meds, but still earned me another trip to the hospital – but just for observation, tests and some lab work. While Barbara and I were there, we met a wonderful woman named Sharon. She was recovering from bypass surgery and needed to get checked out because of some post-operative issues she was having.

We struck up a conversation. Sharon, wrapped up in four blankets, said something about going back into surgery and being scared and nervous. I turned to her and asked, "Do you want us to pray with you?" She said yes and held my hand. So, the three of us prayed. It was touching to see her close her eyes, bow her head in affirmation and open her eyes with a sense of thankfulness for that moment. I learned that part of my own healing process was gaining a better understanding of what others are going through. I learned that, whether you are a patient or caregiver, helping others to heal can be very therapeutic. It was for me as a patient, and maybe it can be for others as well. It's another reason for writing this book. The strength of my Faith is indeed getting better and I believe that's having a direct impact on my well-being. One thing for sure is that it means you're never alone. Knowing that God is with you can be very comforting. Maybe prayers can help somebody allay the fear they have – like the fear Sharon surely had returning to the hospital because things weren't going so well. If someone is a little more comforted as a result, it is a good thing.

Now, I can recognize the power of prayer for myself and others because I see there's a comfort and energy attached to it. When I see someone is really hurting, I just say it: "Would you like me to pray for healing with you?" I've done this dozens of times in the hospital during my volunteer days and 19/20 people say "yes." The old Mark would have never had the courage, confidence, or whatever to even ask this question. But now, there's no hesitation. If you believe that prayer can be a significant part of the healing process, and I do, then it can be. If you don't, then you short change yourself from the benefits that prayer offers. Maybe you are already there or may you have to get to a point where you decide to let God in and not continue to shut Him out. Either way, it can help you feel better. After all, He is the greatest Faith Healer of all time.

HOPE, BELIEF, FAITH

I used to believe that no matter the situation, I could control or influence what would happen. Time after time, I made it through the tough times with the belief I could pull myself out of just about anything. That was my egocentric way to look at things and the very reason that kept my religious commitment from the top spot on my priority list. It never occurred to me that maybe God was intervening on my behalf to get me through whatever personal struggle I was having at the time. But when I look back on the incident in the Grand Canyon, at the 5K, on the racquetball court and several other life threatening situations, I realize that a person can't be lucky that many times. More than one of my doctors has told me that I'm lucky to be alive and I've had several people tell me that God must be looking out for me. I'm inclined to agree.

No longer do I leave this area of the 5 F's and its role in healing to chance. Faith seems to come in three stages: hope, belief and faith. All three can be viewed in a religious context, but let's talk about them globally for a moment. The process begins with Hope. Hope is a necessary ingredient and can be very strong. That said, it seems that if you just hope something is going to be, it doesn't come with any action attached. To me that means: I'm not going to do anything about it and I'm not really going to change much. I just hope I get better. Hope without actions and execution is nothing more than a wish. It's not that I don't hope good things will occur. Believe me, I do. I just can't rely on hope alone. Yet, at the same time, the toughest situations require some degree of hope and that's why I see this as the starting point for the rest of the process. For some people, hope might be all they have at that moment. If that's the case, look deeper and contemplate the effects on your well-being. I think there's more.

The stage that follows Hope is Belief. Belief is where I was stuck, because it had always been about believing in myself to get the job done. I had my faith, I just didn't put all my trust in its power as much as others did. I thought it was up to me. What's missing for some people is that they have no faith at all, so they just believe in whatever they find to make them feel good or more comfortable. These days, it's easier than ever to get caught up in what passes itself off as faith. It's so easy that some guy realizes he doesn't want to make pancakes anymore, decides to start up a church in his garage and calls himself a preacher. Then, he finds a few lost souls and BOOM, he's got a flock. As the flock grows, he moves to a strip mall, then a large auditorium. Next thing you know he's on TV making the case for $20 love offerings while smacking people on the forehead in his expensive, custom-made suit with the tie that doesn't match.

I've never been drawn to being a preacher, but I might have been one of the "tell-me-what-I-want-to-hear" folks sitting in the auditorium. Doing what feels good is so much easier than making a true commitment to "believe" in God more so than oneself. And our society does everything it can to focus people on themselves. What's in it for me? is the first question that comes to mind all too often. I'm guilty as well. But, even so I have a better understanding, especially now, that I'm not here just for me.

My compass has always been pretty good. I've got my parents, wife, kids and many religious business associates to thank for that. But my actions and outcomes weren't always tied to Faith or doing things to give glory to Jesus. The distinction comes out of commitment and an unwavering belief in God. For some things, there just isn't an explanation. You just have to take them on Faith, which isn't easy for many people - certainly it wasn't for me. And it's even harder in the secular TV society that seeks to control the way we think and act. The reality is that everybody has "issues." And some have more than others. It took a long time for me to get on the track to commitment, and I've still got a long way to go, even with so many great examples around me, but I'm thankful for where I am and continue to work on my own "belief" every day.

All that said, hope can be lost and belief can be shaken. That's why we need Faith.

ANOTHER SLAP UPSIDE THE HEAD

I received another slap upside the head about eight months after getting diagnosed with Sarcoidosis and having a pacemaker/defibrillator installed in my chest to keep me alive. Since the "it's all about me" mode is hard to escape, I foolishly believed I had <u>survived</u> multiple near-death experiences. I've come to realize that "I" didn't actually survive; I was <u>spared</u>. Being a slow learner, it took me this long to recognize that God had spared my life. I'm only alive because of that, not the stubbornness or inner strength I've relied upon for so long. Heck, God instilled that in me as well. One of my doctors told me I should be dead "10 times over: and really seemed amazed that I'm still around. I guess that God has a bigger plan for me - one that doesn't involve passing away in my sleep or having heart failure at some grocery store while choosing between blueberry or strawberry Pop Tarts™ (neither of which I'm supposed to eat). Here's the thing: I don't know what the plan is for me. It's something I have to pray on and figure out for myself knowing that I'll never be privy to what God's plan actually is. People spend way too much time trying to figure out what God's plan is. But, no one will ever know. You make decisions and move down that path doing the best you can and trying to do the right thing. As best as I've been able to figure out so far, it means I have to be on the lookout for opportunities to give thanks, serve others, give back and get better spiritually. I think God wants me to tell you how rekindling my faith is helping me not only to get better, but to "be" better. And it's never too late. When I'm delivering Communion to patients at the hospital, I often meet people that tell me they haven't been to church for 15 years. It's amazing how many times they want me to stay and pray with them. I think deep down they want to come back to know God, but they're just in the habit of thinking that they're not good enough, or that it doesn't matter. Well it does matter. If you've been given a second chance at life or if you're just hanging on, you can still change everything. Maybe prayer is one way to come to a closer understanding about the role faith can play in your own healing process. Try it. You might find some consolation, comfort and inner strength there. And that cannot be a bad thing.

My wife goes to church about three or four times per week and spends at least an hour every week in an Adoration Chapel. Her father passed away not too long ago. He was a kind and gentle man who was unbelievably devout and unwavering in his belief. Wow, Grandpa B knew exactly what he was about, where he was going, and what he believed. There was no doubt in his mind because everything he did was Faith based. He was strong. Looking at him you'd think: I'll never be that devout. How do I get there? I've tried to be a good example, but my late father-in-law still leads in this category. He's been a spiritual role model for my wife, kids and for me as well.

Ever since the kids were born, I started to ask those questions. I was in my 40's before I really began to reflect on strengthening my Faith. Everything continually came back to how committed and willing to change I was. I've got a lot of work to do in terms of developing my Faith to be as strong as my wife and kids. They are truly committed. My Faith journey is a work in progress, but I can't imagine not having any Faith at all. I know of a man who had succeeded in everything he'd done. His self-confidence was overwhelming. When he got ill and continued to get worse, he experienced depression for the first time in his life. He had always been able to meet every challenge because of his belief in himself. He even took pride in being a "self-made" millionaire. But no one is self-made. It's not possible. It takes other people to teach you what you need to know and help you achieve what you set out to achieve. Now, he is losing the fight for his life and for the first time, there's nothing he can do about it. Since he has no faith - no belief in God, he has no reserve to draw from - no higher source to put his belief in. It's still all about him and he can't believe it's playing out this way. He is losing hope because he has no belief aside from himself and that well has run dry. He is to the point of giving up because he won't let God in to comfort him and give him a new form of strength that he never had. That could be me, but thankfully it's not. I "decided" to let go and have Faith.

So, hope and prayer can lead to belief. Then next stage in the progression is when your belief fuels your Faith. I've traveled around the Earth for 50 plus years without a total level of commitment to my Faith. I'm fortunate now to have found that strength in Him and it is truly powerful. I believe. Now, I've got to sign on the line and move forward.

I relied heavily on faith in the 10 months before my collapse when they couldn't figure out what was wrong with me. I just wasn't getting any better. In fact, I was getting worse. Then we learned my situation was even more serious than we initially imagined. I know that I can't hope my way through some of the health challenges I'll face…it will take a measured dosage of belief and faith.

Again, I'm not trying to convert anyone here. All I can do is relate my own experience. You can't just cross your fingers and wait for tomorrow, "hoping" it will be better. I've learned that faith in God gives me the belief that I am going to get better and the strength to handle things if I don't - which is equally important. Maybe you are experiencing this already…or maybe you want to.

Let's face it, once we get tagged as a "patient," nothing is business as usual anymore. The old mindset that put me, myself and I out front on the list of my top three priorities has been wiped out. I temporarily stepped down as the president of my company. I resigned as the executive director of the association I started. I gave up managing my soccer team and odds at that moment in time weren't in my favor that I'll ever return to play the game I love, or ever be able to go for a long run with my kids. When everything changes, you have to find the silver lining. I'm working to make "Faith in God" No. 1 on my list, even though I managed to avoid making Him the priority for so many years. I never lived my faith before. I'm trying to live it now by being thankful for every day and looking for opportunities to brighten someone else's day. I was surprised to find how many people in my work world would pray with me. I think that my illness has given me strength, belief and a greater understanding of my purpose. It's a tough way to get the message, but now that I've been given multiple chances to get it right, maybe I will.

Maybe you are a caregiver and can help someone who needs to find comfort in God. And, as I've learned during this process, Faith helps healing. God bless you.

WHY ME? ... WHY NOT ME?

Medically speaking, there's no reason why I should be here. Apparently, I'm one of those anomalies that happen where there's no reason for me to have contracted this disease other than the obvious – I won the Bad Health Lottery. This will make the next sentence sound really weird – I'm thankful that it happened to me. Not glad, not overjoyed, not at all happy it happened to me, but thankful. First of all, I'm thankful it didn't happen to my kids, my wife or my extended family. As I've mentioned, it's also helping me understand my Faith a lot more. Early on in my illness, right after one of my many doctor's appointments, I flipped on the radio in my wife's car and Catholic Family Radio was on the dial. Just by coincidence (or maybe not), there was a priest talking about his own illness and he helped me realize it does no good to ask "Why me?" but rather we should ask, "Why not me?" It is what it is. You have to take what comes and make the best of the situation – for yourself and those around you. There's a line at the end of the Tom Hanks' movie "Saving Private Ryan" where his character is dying and says to Private Ryan: *"Earn this."* What he means is that Ryan needs to seize upon the opportunity to live the best life he can after all that was done to rescue him. I think about that line because of all that was done to rescue me...physically and spiritually. I'm still here. I was spared for some reason, and I now have the opportunity to try to earn this every day. So, if you're able to read this, be thankful for that and think about what you can do with today.

BACK TO THE CANYON

Let's go back to where this all began: the Grand Canyon.

Every time I go to the canyon I am struck with a sense of reverence. In the Canyon, there's no doubt in my mind that God exists. You look at this vast expanse of incredible beauty and wonder how this could be created without God's hand. It's just unbelievable. You look around and a feeling comes over you to where all you can say is: "Wow, well done here." Hard as it might be to believe, I don't think God tests us — even if His plan includes climbing out of His glorious creation with a dangerous heart condition. Instead, He gives you a series of opportunities that we can choose to learn from or not. It took me a long time to understand this and learn from the health predicaments I find myself in.

Many of you may have also had multiple close calls, misdiagnosis, ups, downs, endless tests and bottles full of meds, and may still face some rough sledding ahead. For some reason, you made it through so far. In my case, God must be up there saying, "Alright, listen. You're going to have to get through all this stuff to get to the answer because you still don't get it. It's not about you." I'll bet He looked at St. Peter and said, "Geez, this Landiak dude is awfully dense." St. Peter no doubt replied, "Should I slap him upside the head again to get his attention?"

Sitting in that hospital bed, I started to think about how to "earn" my extra time on this earth. In business, my job is to consult and drive people to action. Now, as a patient, I'm drawn to do service in an effort to give "something" back. I'm both a patient and a volunteer at the hospital that 10 years ago hired me to teach them about customer service in a healthcare environment. That's ironic, isn't it? Now, I'm one of their best customers.

Would I have done some of the things I'm doing now 10 years ago? I doubt it. The thoughts behind those actions have been with me all along; I'm just now acting upon them for the first time. I'm far from perfect and Lord knows I have a long way to go. Maybe you want to come with me? Who knows, maybe I was supposed to write this book so you could read it and be inspired to get better in some aspect of your life. If that's the case, drop me a line and let me know. I feel fortunate to have talked with so many people who have inspired me to press on in the best way possible with each new day. Who inspires you?

"THERE AIN'T NO ATHEISTS ON TURBULENT AIRCRAFT"

I remember watching "The Tonight Show" years ago when host Johnny Carson did an interview with comedian Buddy Hackett, a guy who had a unique form of comedy that always cracked me up. Hackett was quite the storyteller and always told his tales "in the rough." His delivery wasn't dirty (ok, sometimes it was), just unpolished. Hackett had a quick wit and did comedy off the cuff. During this particular interview, Hackett was talking about flying in a particularly rough storm when he blurts out, "Ya know Johnny, there ain't no atheists on turbulent aircraft." The same could be said for the ICU. Everyone on the floor is, or was at one point, fighting to survive, which means there's a lot of first-time praying going on from patients, family and friends. That's not to say this is the first time these people have ever said a few words to God, but it might be that now the conversation had a real purpose or passion behind it. The conversation was real.

If you choose to use your situation – as a patient, loved one or caregiver – to grow stronger in your Faith, you will. It also helps to know there will be so many people who will help you along the way because of their own Faith. A pastor, priest, rabbi, family member or friend would be more than happy to discuss God with you. Here's the thing: regardless of your level of belief, talking with clergy or others who have God in their lives might just bring you some comfort, which is a very good thing.

Hospitals also create a tremendous amount of apprehension for friends and family. (About this time, if you're the patient, you're thinking: "what about the apprehension I'm feeling?) Your closest friend in the world might stay away from visiting to avoid seeing you all hooked up to machines, in some level of discomfort and/or full of meds you don't want to be taking. In the realm of Faith, some people might be too uncomfortable to bring up God and spirituality simply because they don't know your feelings or because they think it's taboo. The average person won't just walk in and ask to pray with you. While many times the answer will be yes, it's the simple act of asking that should make everyone involved feel a little better. Maybe your physical health will improve, and it will for sure help with your mental fitness which is also so very important.

Having a visitor join you in saying grace before a hospital meal is another way of showing them it's OK to pray with or for you. And, it's so easy and natural to do. Adding the healing elements into saying grace makes it about more than just the food. And, when you're in the hospital, let's face it, the food is something that probably needs a prayer too.

An item that brought me great comfort was a crucifix that Mary, one of my wife's best friends, had bought for me when she was visiting Medjugorje, a small town in western Bosnia and Herzegovina, where the Virgin Mary is said to have appeared on multiple occasions. I had always carried it in my briefcase while traveling, and I placed it on my tray table in the hospital. It was interesting how many people recognized and commented on it. They would take notice of it and it almost immediately got us into a conversation. "Yeah, that's my strength," I would say if someone spotted the crucifix. Next thing you know, we're having a Faith conversation. Having the cross present let people know that Faith was something we could talk about and share. Not just with family and friends, but it worked with the nurses, food delivery people and others, as well. To this day, I always keep it close. (Thanks Mary)

If you are open to allowing Faith to be part of your healing process, it can do some good. There's no guarantee in anything, especially since so much is out of your control. Having Faith makes it easier...not easy – just easier. The healing process is different for everyone and there are times when you might want to give up. But, I'm convinced that God may have something for you to do. For those of us living on borrowed time to begin with, He's only going to allow so much time for us to do it. Time to get to work getting better.

THIS IS YOUR LENT

The season of Lent is the most holy time of the year for Christians. It marks Jesus's 40-day retreat into the desert, and serves as a period of reflection and sacrifice leading up to Easter when Christ rose from the dead after being tortured and crucified. For some, it has become a reason for many to give up sweets or some other indulgence in the hopes of dropping a few pounds. For others, it is a time for growth. Aside from giving up some of the basics, I never did anything extraordinary during Lent, except for my collapse outside the racquetball court and subsequent trip to the ICU.

The timing of my illness was not lost on Father Pat, who told me when I was in the Intensive Care Unit that, "This is your Lent." Of course, I joked back, saying, "Actually Father, I was thinking of giving up potato chips or cookies, not dealing with a major heart disorder." All kidding aside, what he said was so powerful to me. Sure, it's easy to get caught up in all the things I've had to "give up" – running, soccer, work, my lifestyle and just feeling "normal." I was having to come to grips with the fact that my new normal, my Lent, was about learning from the sacrifice of giving up all the things I could no longer do and how to adapt to being sick. It helped me to see another aspect of what Lent is all about – the idea of reflection on where we are with our Faith. It seems this is an ongoing process. That's where I'm at. I'm still learning what getting better in my Faith means.

All of this comes back to the healing process in a simple way. The stronger one's faith is, the more at peace you can be with what is happening to you. Instead of asking "Why me?," we can choose to be more thankful for what we have. That's because we can always find other folks who have greater obstacles to overcome. The guy checking in people for lab work on the day I met Sharon was in a wheelchair. He had no legs. He proved to be as pleasant a person as you'd ever want to meet. Wow, that's amazing to me. My problems seem to pale in comparison. I have what I have, but I can still get up and walk across the room every day. Look what this guy has to deal with. Still, he's learned how to come to terms with his disability and go on living with a smile on his face. I don't know if he is a man of faith, but he is a man of tremendous inner strength and that's got to come from someplace other than his own ego.

Right now, I'm in a life-altering stage. Things have changed dramatically, but life altering might mean there may be a silver lining inside the clouds. To see only the negatives in life-altering events robs from your ability to heal. While my physical being fights to recuperate and heal, I'm altering other parts of my life to be a better person and maybe that can bring out the best in others. My journey has gone from a near-death experience to a "nearer-to-life" experience. With a stronger Faith, maybe yours can, too.

ANSWERING "*THAT*" QUESTION

When you've been in the hospital for a few days, you look haggard. When you've had a procedure or two, and have been there a week or more, you look like you've been living on the streets. The most obvious time people truly understood my situation came during my hospital stays. In a hospital bed, unshaven with greasy, disheveled hair, hooked up to monitors, I was completely out of context to family, friends and those who know me through business. It became my goal to set the tone for those visits in a way that didn't have people walking out of there thinking about how glad they were not to be the poor S.O.B. stuck in that hospital bed (although they probably thought it anyway).

Undoubtedly, the first question to pop out from everyone was, and still is, "How are you doing?" It became apparent very quickly that how you answer this question sets up the rest of the conversation and can impact their entire visit, if not your entire day. I've developed an arsenal of replies to this question that I can tailor to the individual. One favorite is: "I'm getting better every day." This means something to whomever it is you are talking with. It makes them go, "Oh, good," when they've probably prepared to hear bad news because they know you are sick. Am I actually getting better? That depends on how you look at it. Medically, during some periods, maybe not. But when you frame it around the overall picture, there's always some facet of your life that might be getting better. Whether it's becoming stronger in Faith, building a better relationship with family members and friends, enjoying your surroundings more, getting stronger mentally or just treating people differently, the response works. The answer doesn't always have to be about your physical being. The answer to how you are doing can be framed in the context of you as a whole person, not just about your ailment. That mindset has become more prevalent since I left the hospital. With my friends, I can respond with a smart ass remark that will let them know that my sense of humor is still intact. For example, here are some of the other responses you can use to answer *that* question:

So, how are you doing?

"As of today, I'm not in a hospital bed or prison, so you gotta like that."

To borrow a line from Caddy Shack: "Well the Dali Lama says I'll receive total consciousness on my death bed...so I've got that going for me."

"My horoscope says there is a specter of goodness surrounding my orb."

"If I were any better, my meds would be taking me."

"I feel like a million bucks. The ones that get shot by hunters and hit by cars."

"Let's not go there. How are you doing?"

"Look at the monitor behind me. If the lines are still going up and down, I'm doing great."

"Well let's just say that I'm on the right side of the dirt."

"If you don't count any of the stuff that's happened in the last several years, I am fantastic."

"Well my nurse told me that having a bowel movement is a good sign, so as of this morning, I'm good."

"Ask me tomorrow. If I'm still here, then today I'm doing OK."

"Yep."

"I'm somewhere between needing a nap and not completely unwell."

"Well I'm heavily medicated and not currently in a position to answer that question."

"Oh, let's just say the Lord's plan is fully in place."

"My cardiologist advised me to avoid additional stress and not answer that question."

"Have you ever downed a pint of rat poison or been hit in the head with a hammer?"

"Geez if I was any better they'd have to bronze a statue of me and put it in my front yard."

"I'll tell you…if you can explain to me what: "you have an acute myocardial infarction of the reperfusion type where the infarct is diffusely hemorrhagic," means."

YOU LOOK GREAT!

One of the common complaints that sarco's have is that the disease tears you apart on the inside, so you can look good on the outside, but feel horrific. A big part of this is the disease itself, but much of it is also from the meds used to treat the disease. These are the dreaded "side effects." My fellow Sarcoidosis patients, and maybe some of you, often suffer from: intense pain, difficulty moving, intense fatigue, inability to breathe, weight gain, migraines, feeling sick to our stomach 24/7, or the 100+ other side orders that come with a medicinal meal. Whether you are a heart or cancer patient, or been in an accident or have some other odd malady, you can probably relate to some of these new facts of life.

Back in my natural elements, the how-are-you-feeling conversations didn't slow down. People saw me up and around, at home functioning, doing some of my job, *looking* more like my old self. The kids see me laughing and smiling around the dinner table, and probably figure Dad's doing better. Things appear more normalized because aside from some visual changes due to the meds, I look OK on the outside. People don't realize how you actually feel, what's going on internally or that you may have a very long way to go. It's at that point that we have to decide how to project ourselves while we heal. Being incapacitated in the hospital is very different than everyday life at home, so it becomes even more important to decide how you want to present yourself and your situation. People want you to be better, it's just that they don't know how they can help you do it. So, I decided it's my job to set the mood for these interactions.

Maybe you actually do look a lot better on the outside and that's great. People don't know about all the tests you underwent that failed to provide any idea of what was wrong inside you and the ongoing search for answers — they can't see how you feel on the inside and that's fine. If someone asks a more specific question, I'll tell them the abridged medical version of my condition. But most often, when I meet people or see my friends, I don't really want to talk about my illness. A friend asked me to breakfast and opened up wanting to know how I was doing. I gave him one of my more subtle prepared responses and then immediately turned it around and asked him, "How's your kid?" For the next 30 minutes we talked about his family, work and sports. That's so much more interesting than talking about the recent adjustments to my pacemaker. It's an example of how my focus has changed. I'm looking for more opportunities to ask questions, listen, and learn more about the other person. This is a bit of a change for me as I seemed always to be in high gear and rarely took the time before. My willingness and desire to spend more time getting to know the other person has grown and made for much more interesting conversations.

While people now look at my exterior to see a more healthy-looking Mark, I'm looking deeper to understand what's happening with them. It's a choreographed dance, one I'll choose every time over a conversation about irregular heart rhythms and nausea. I'm always looking for an opportunity to feel better; and not focusing on my illness is one way. One of my walking buddies, Gary, and I have known each other for 15 years as soccer friends. I definitely put him on the "good guys" list. For quite some time, he joined me almost every week for a 40-minute stroll around the neighborhood. We'd get the obligatory "So, how you doin'?" question out of the way quickly. Conversations don't dwell too much on what's wrong with me, or on the health issue he's recovering from. It's just two guys walking and talking. After about three weeks, I realized, as I did with my friend Ted, that I knew more about Gary through these walks than I did after all the years we played soccer together. He agrees. These interactions with Gary have made me better in the friend category because our relationship strengthened. It just feels better to be around people that can take your mind off the rough stuff. And that diversion is part of the mental fitness and mental toughness you have to work on throughout the healing process. Your mind, in turn, helps drive the physical fitness of recovery. During the writing of this book, Gary was informed that they found spots on his liver and back. It turned out to be cancerous and he had to go through chemo drip therapies and skin grafts to treat it. It was a shift in roles. Now I was the supporter and he was the patient in trouble. Talking about health issues with someone who is also having health issues is different. You understand each other's circumstances and can play an important support role for one another. Reversing the roles and becoming the supporter meant putting my own ideas into action. How could I help this person best utilize the 5 F's in their upcoming procedures and subsequent recovery? Maybe you know someone having some serious health issues. If you are the friend, family member or caregiver, here are some ways to use some of the 5F's to support the patient:

- Faith: What role does Faith play in this person's life, and could you offer to pray with, or at least let them know you'll be praying for them? Do they need a ride to church?

- Family: Are you family? What support role can you provide? Should you "just show up?"

- Friends: What support can you, as a friend offer? (Visits? Exercise? Rides? Phone Calls? Send notes/books? Research? Meals? Positive Reinforcement, Etc.)

- Fitness: What can you do to help the person prepare mentally and physically for what is to come? (Offer positive reinforcement, help them to stretch, walk or exercise to the best of their ability)?

- Fun: What types of activities, antics, stories, jokes, games, etc. could you surprise them with that would bring a distraction or an element of normalcy and fun to the day?

LET'S TALK FITNESS

Now that we've talked about Family, Friends and Faith at some length, let's talk about Fitness. I talked with Gary about "going in strong" (to the 10 days of treatments) both mentally and physically. I've found that both mental and physical preparation are essential. Mental preparation helps you deal with the anxiety and stress that can accompany surgery or serious illness, and recovery. Physical preparation means getting your body in the best shape you can to deal with the actual surgeries, recovery and/or minimize the side effects that med treatments can bring.

FITNESS 101: "YOU GOTTA FEED THE ENGINE"

When Gary had to go into the hospital, people were great about bringing food over, so his wife Becky wouldn't have to cook. This is a great way to help the family out if you're looking for how you can help and have the ability to cook a tasty and healthy meal. I told him the story of my dad who always tells us how important it is to "feed the engine" whenever you're sick.

You need to eat what you can to keep your body working at it's best. Here are 10 pieces of advice I've cobbled together from the recommendations of friends, family and physicians. But first, my disclaimer: 1) Don't eat what your doc tells you not to, and, 2) I don't know if any of this works...but it sounds reasonable.

1. Eat some fresh fruits, vegetables and berries every day (especially these "power" foods: cherries, kiwi, watermelon, cantaloupe, guava, beans, watercress, kale, spinach, onions, carrots, cabbage and broccoli)...and the fresher the better. OK, so you hated many of these as a kid and made it through childhood just fine. Now they're supposed to be good for you...so make yourself a smoothie.

2. Drink plenty of water – Some water guru's tell us to drink 8, 8-oz glasses/day). Who does this? Only people

who are always close to a bathroom. For some of us, water is a balancing act. Talk to your doctor about volumes especially if you're taking diuretics and running to the rest room 30 seconds after any liquid intake.

3. Stay away from soda, high-salt snacks, high-fat foods, snacks and deserts with high sugar content and high-cholesterol foods. In other words, don't eat anything you really like.

4. If you're supposed to take your meds with food, take 'em with food. (I like to take mine with all the items in #3)

5. Cook w/ olive or coconut oil instead of butter or grease and when a recipe calls for sugar, cut the quantity in half. Better yet, let someone else cook

6. Eat smaller portions if you are overweight and take seconds if you look emaciated.

7. Ask your doctor about vitamins and supplements before you purchase $1000 worth of pills from a late night infomercial.

8. Eat fish at least once a week (especially salmon, mackerel, bluefish which are high in Omega 3). Or if you hate fish, just eat a bowl of Omega 3.

9. Substitute a salad or veggies for French fries if you're having a burger or steak. Yes, it's ok to have red meat on occasion, just in case you thought I was trying to convert you to vegetarianism after reading item #1. Like my friend Mike says: "If God didn't want us to eat meat, he wouldn't have made it taste so good."

10. And this is my favorite piece of advice given to me by a doctor: "Eat whatever you want…just do it in moderation." I love this guy. (Please pass the bag of Cheetos)

MENTAL TOUGHNESS

One of my business mentors used to tell me to "expect the best, but prepare for the worst." Everyone wants to get better and is hoping to hear good news from their doctors, but sometimes the news is bad. I know that negative news is one of the potential outcomes for me and have mentally braced myself in case that's the result. I prepare myself by doing some research on the potential outcomes and creating a list of questions to ask the doctor.

Almost every doctor I've seen has told me that having the right mindset helps the healing process significantly. Having a positive frame of mind is easier for some than others. My son works with a foreign gentlemen who describes difficult situations with this phrase: "easy for say...not so easy for do." That's become pretty popular around our house and it rings true for people facing difficult health scenarios. Fear, uncertainty, anxiety, and doubt are all powerful emotions and can erode our confidence, attitude and outlook. Like its partner, physical fitness, we have to work on our mental fitness every day if we want it be in the best shape possible for taking on obstacles. It is an important and necessary component to our well-being. And, then there's the mental prep necessary to handle the compromising moments that healing presents.

HEALING, HUMILITY
AND HUMILIATION

As patients, we need to be aware that some of the facets of getting better are difficult to prepare for. Among them is the fact that at times, healing can be humbling, and even humiliating. This is another one of the many realities among the mental challenges we face.

Aside from the beat up, combed your hair with a pork chop look, med loopiness, dozing off mid-sentence and need for help with simple tasks, there's the other dreaded "side effects." My rheumatologist referred me to a dermatologist who is familiar with my disease to check for signs of it on my skin. I have a few epidermal issues, but the worries were a nasty rash on my ankle, hip and buttocks. And where did the rash decide to wreak havoc? On my butt, of course.

This might all sound like a common referral until I tell you that I was sent to a doctor at a well-known teaching hospital. Still not a big deal, right? Well, I get in the exam room and a 23 year old med student who fits the image of what you'd expect Pamela Anderson's daughter to look like walks in. Her name is Michelle, but I prefer to think in terms of her stage name: Sunshine. So, Sunshine takes my history and in the first of many uncomfortable moments to come, she has me strip and put on one of those high-fashion, pastel hospital aprons with little guppies printed on it. Of course, you have to put it on backwards. And, even after 200 or so practice opportunities, I still can't seem to get the damn things tied properly. This is even more frustrating because there is enough string on this enormous paper towel to rappel out the window to the ground five stories below - which I should have done right then. Too late. There's a knock at the door and she reappears to gather in the sight of my bowed legs protruding from the bottom of my new wardrobe item just as I finish tying off the last of the tentacles.

In one of life's most humbling moments, Sunshine checks out the rash on my ankle and hip and then starts evaluating the painfully itchy redness on my rash-covered butt. As she does this, I can't help thinking: "I have socks older than you." It gets worse – the exam, not the rash. After hanging out behind me for an eternity, Sunshine calls in the "assistant." In walks a Czechoslovakian MD in training named Olga, who asks me a few questions in heavily accented English about my sarcoidosis. She starts to examine my arms, legs and ankles and then - BOTH OF THEM get behind me. Sunshine and Olga spread the back of my apron like a curtain at the theatre and start discussing the possible causes of the mystery rash on the back end of my carcass. "Vat you tink dis iz?" she asks Sunshine. There must've been a movie playing out my back end because they lingered there for what seemed like about 90 minutes. When the show was over, they closed the curtain and both left the room saying "the specialist" – apparently the doc with the most butt-rash experience – would be with me "in a moment."

I'm sure the conversation outside the room went something like this:

"Well doctor, this guy is one step away from total heart failure, but you've GOT to see the rash on his cheeks. And we're not talking about his face."

Now comes the MOST humbling moment.

With Sunshine and Olga following along in order of seniority, in marches the Queen of Dermatology, who goes through the same Q&A routine as the resident trainee. Then, all three of them waltz around behind me as the good doctor starts a full-length lecture on possible causes of ass rashes in immune-compromised patients; all the while I'm feeling a draft behind me. Now comes the ultimate humiliation. The Queen then asks Olga to "take a culture." This is Derma Code for sticking a Q-tip® between your cheeks and moving it around like you're mixing a cocktail.

I'm usually pretty good about coming up with something whimsical to say to break the ice during magical moments like these. However, it appears there is a nerve in your rear end, that when pressed with a Q-tip®, turns off your brain and paralyzes your face with a blank, stunned look on it. With this ordeal now behind me (pun intended), I had to face the trio while Dr. B (as in Butt rash) tells me everything to do for my skin maladies. What an ordeal. If I had it to do all over again, I'd rather sit in a pool of alcohol and light my bottom on fire. Sure, it would cause some minor burns, but I think the scorch-and-burn treatment would clear up the rash and avoid yet another episode in Mark's most humiliating medical moments.

The lesson here is, well, actually there is no lesson here.

Maybe we just have to leave it at the idea that you have to prepare your mind to deal with the side effects that come with the healing process. Not just the rashes, sickness, aches and pains, but, being humbled and humiliated at times during the process. I guess one positive outcome is that none of them could pick me out of a line up.

HEY, GET OUT OF THAT BED

Now, some might say you are a pretty self-driven person, but some doctors are even more driven than you are. When Dr. Greenstein visited me in my room a few hours after slitting my chest and inserting a defibrillator and several wires running into my heart, he gave me a directive. "Get out of the bed. We need to get you up and moving as soon as possible." It was only a few hours out of surgery and I must admit that laying there for a while and catching some sleep sounded much more appealing. I've been active my entire life and right up to the onset of my illness, I spent years sprinting up and down a soccer field. I wasn't really very skilled, but I could always run pretty fast up until my illness hit. Now all that had changed. Goal #1 was get my feet on the floor. Doing so was as much a mental task as a physical one. Can your head force your body to do something it doesn't really want to do? Judging by the divorce rate in this country, yes, but that doesn't have anything to do with this conversation. The point is that it is SO much easier to stay in bed, take a nap or use your illness to mentally justify a lack of activity and limit your mobility.

How do you set your head in these difficult moments when fear is the natural reaction? A lot of people are fearful and scared of what's going to happen or what could happen. Worry is a separate issue. While I didn't have much fear, I have worried that my wife won't have her husband and my kids won't have their dad. Worry causes stress and stress is no good for healing. In fact it has just the opposite effect. On another level, I still think (not worry): what if I won't ever be able to hike the Grand Canyon again or do some of the other things I love. I worry, but I'm not afraid I won't be able to do them. It can be difficult to discern and separate fear and worry, so channeling away those feelings becomes important. Fear and worry become misdirected energy that distract from healing. All your focus should be on getting better. Too many people want to figure out what's going to happen next. Instead, think about what you could do right now and put together an idea of what you'd like to have happen as your goal for the day, week, month or year. At that very moment, I wasn't sure that I could get out of bed. But, I did…and I stepped ever so cautiously the two feet to the chair next to the bed and sat down. "Good. That's your first step. Next try to go a couple more steps and see how it feels. If you're awake, stay out of the bed." OK, there was the old adage in action. A journey of 1,000 miles begins with a single step. And so it was for me on March 1st, 2012. My first step toward a better quality of life 1000 miles away. I wasn't sure I could do it, but when I took that step, it was euphoric. I didn't know what that meant for me and my family at that point, but now that I knew the first step was possible and since it didn't kill me, I was ready and willing to give it my all to find out. My docs and I built a 5-year plan once we knew what we were up against. I'm naturally impatient, so ratcheting back my expectations for getting better by 5 years required some realignment of my thinking.

Here's a tip for all of us: ***You are stronger than you think you are.***

Dr. Greenstein told my friend Dan that I'm very determined to beat the odds. That's true. I don't want to go backwards to where I was. Been there. Done that. Hated it.

For me, the ultimate was a return to the soccer field with my team, the ability to run with my kids, or simply go for a walk with my wife in the forest preserve or on a beach. What can I do today to bring myself a little closer to that destination? I try to accomplish something every day, even little things – anything I can put in the WIN column. Every small win can make a big difference. Physical battles are one thing, but, in many ways, the mental fights are the toughest to win. The mental struggle wages on when it comes to treatment and recovery after your trip to the hospital. Some of those battles are more aggravating than painful. Sleep Apnea is one of those battles.

MY NIGHT AT THE SLEEP CLINIC

Part of the lengthy diagnosis process for me involved a visit to the sleep clinic to check for Sleep Apnea, which, as it turns out, I was able to add to my list of maladies that had been aggravating my condition. I was diagnosed with a condition called Cheyne-Stokes Apnea which they tell me can kill you in your sleep if not treated - especially if you're a heart patient. So off I go to the Sleep Clinic for evaluation. The name for this place is a ruse. Instead of "Sleep Clinic" it should be called the "YOU'RE NOT GOING TO GET ANY SLEEP CLINIC." My first visit started around 9 p.m. when I was met by a heavily muscled technician I'll call Brutus. They start off by putting you in a very nice bedroom with cameras suitable for making unsuitable home movies. The lights were so bright I had to rub a little SPF 75 on my face to prevent sunburn. At this point, I'm pretty sure they only make the video as a way to threaten a worldwide YouTube broadcast of you snoring just in case you don't pay your bill on time.

Next, you fill out forms as long as the Federal Tax Code which essentially seeks information they should already have. Perhaps reading these 67,000 pages will help you fall asleep, <u>but that's not going to happen</u> because Brutus has arrived with a cart filled with enough wires to redo the electrical system in the Empire State Building (see picture on back cover). After an hour of placing and testing electrodes on my head and upper chest, I now resemble Lady Gaga on a bad day. I'm completely exhausted and ready to pass out, <u>but that's not going to happen</u>

because it's time to get fitted for the CPAP mask – think of a bulkier, more obtrusive, Darth Vader set up – that shoves air in your nose and mouth in a manner unlike the way any human breathes. Six mask-fitting attempts, and many minutes later, Brutus finally found a mask not leaking any air from it.

I'm now beyond exhaustion and can't wait to sleep, <u>but that's not going to happen</u> because it's time to do an in-bed version of the P90X fitness program and play the Sleep Clinic edition of Jeopardy, so they can check all their equipment. Finally, Brutus gives the good-to-go sign, and the interrogation lamps are turned off. Despite the lamps, the room up to this point has been arctic cold and the heat is now turned on to avoid the inevitable frostbite. Brutus now has the audacity to tell me it's time to sleep, <u>but that's not going to happen</u> because I'm covered in wires, wearing a fighter pilot mask and completely awake from the recent interview and pseudo-Jazzercise routine. It feels more like time to grab some OJ and the morning paper. I tell Brutus, viewing me on camera from another room, that I'm not tired. Being the trained professional that he was, he offered me this sound advice, "You really need to go to sleep." Unimpressed and aggravated, I thought to myself, "You really need to go to …."

I have no idea what time it was, but I've probably dozed off for less time than a fraternity pledge gets to sleep in his burlap underwear during initiation week, when Brutus barges in, turns on the light, and says my mask is leaking and needs adjusting. Despite my orders for him to turn off the light and leave, Brutus tightens my facial apparatus to the point where my eyes are bugging out and I can't feel my ears. Fifteen minutes later, I summon Brutus back to unhook me, so I can take the middle of the night trip to the bathroom most men over 50 are all too familiar with. Semi-conscious and unfamiliar with the surroundings, I stumble toward the pitch black relief room covered in wires and incoherently pee on the trash can next to the toilet.

The next thing I know, Brutus is waking me. He says it's 5 a.m. and the test is over. I tell him to get out and come back at 8. Again, he is not amused and tells me to shower and wash my hair to clean out the gunk used to attach the electrodes. Problem is, this appears to be the same epoxy-like stuff also used to hold together the space shuttle and it does not come out easily. Cleaned up, dressed and now bald, I see Brutus once again. He asks if I have any questions. Silly me, I posed four different queries about the test. He replied with exactly the same response each time, "I can't answer that, as the doctor has to interpret the results." After my fourth attempt, he actually had the nerve to ask, "Did you have any _other_ questions?" Astonished, I used my best smart-aleck voice to ask: "Perhaps you can tell me what time the IHOP down the street opens for breakfast, or do I need to ask my doctor?" With a dirty look, Brutus sent me on my way.

The mask was a part of my regular "sleep" routine for just over 4 years. When I got fitted for the home version, the technician actually asked whether I was excited to get it. I said, "Yeah, I can't wait to sleep less. I can't wait to look like the Elephant Man and keep my wife from sleeping due to the noise. I am so psyched about that." What kind of a question was that, anyway? Who wants to wear one of these things? Unrelenting, he countered by trying to sell me visions of a better night's sleep. "Are you kidding me? A better night's sleep? To my knowledge, I'm not having trouble sleeping now despite you telling me that I wake up 29 times per hour and snore like a walrus. When you give me this thing, that's when I'm going to have trouble sleeping."

Mentally, I had to gear up every night to put the stupid mask on. I didn't want to strap this contraption on so tight so that it actually works the way it is supposed to, but I did. It was one of the least favorite treatments that I had to do. I'd rather go back to my IV drip treatments or eat a bowl of maggots (the latter of which was not one of my treatments). Every night I had to prepare my mind for the reality that when I'm most tired at the end of the day, when I really want to go to sleep, I have to put a loud, obnoxious octopus on my face and call it a day. The good news is that about 1,100 days after that initial donning of the mask, I passed the re-test and got to put it on the shelf. Chances are good that I may have to wear it again someday. But for now, it's another small victory in the battle to get better.

Understanding my limitations wasn't bad, it just acted as a mile marker of where I'm at in the battle and a reminder to live within the limits. The mental fitness part of recovery is about where you are right now and where the next step will take you, even if each step is a baby step. If you're the patient, I'm sure that you have some elements of your ailment, your procedures and your ongoing treatment plan that require mental preparation and toughness. Humor and humility help for sure. Faith comes into play as well. Maybe bring a family member or friend along with you for moral support. Which of the 5 elements can you deploy to help you cope with everything you will face or are facing? If you are the caregiver, this can be an emotional time and you need to keep it together as well. Trying to keep things light, staying positive and providing ongoing encouragement can help with both the patient's mental state and that of your own.

One thing is sure for all of us patients, we're not going to transport ourselves forward or back by wishing. I'd love to be two years further into my recovery, but I have to cope as best I can in this moment and prepare for what's to come. You do as well. So, would you mind handing me that facial breathing apparatus and commenting on how young it makes me look?

OH, MY ACHING BACK

The thought of what I can and can't do frequently pops into my head, especially when I'm talking to the doctors. For so long, I didn't know what I was facing, and it's really difficult to defeat an enemy when you don't know what it is, what you're up against, or how to fight it. That can certainly work against a positive outlook. Sometimes, your doctors don't know exactly how to fight it either. There are protocols for this and for that, but every patient is different and sometimes the protocols need to be tweaked to fit the patient. Here's another thing I learned: Find a doctor who is willing to tweak your protocol to find a solution. I know two doctors who came to a very quick judgment and gave up on me before we even started a program for getting better. Years before getting sick, I hurt my back very badly. I was driving home after a meeting with my chiropractor when a kid who thought he was a part of Jeff Gordon's race team, decided to make a left turn from the right lane and hit the gas to beat the oncoming traffic — except he realized he wasn't going to make it and stopped right in front me. He never looked. BANG. We collided going about 40 mph and it gave me one heck of a jolt — to the point where my back hurt so badly I couldn't get out of the car. I was already having severe back problems at the time and this crash happened not even 10 minutes after leaving the chiropractor's office. It was the epitome of temporary relief.

Nothing was broken, but the accident left me with painful back spasms. I could barely walk, and getting out of a chair caused excruciating discomfort. My first doc didn't think it could be fixed, and said this meant no more golf, tennis or racquetball. Deciding not to accept his assessment, I found another doctor. But, he told me the same thing. Neither one explored options with me about what might be possible. I was about to accept their diagnosis – at least temporarily. But, a neighbor told me about a doctor that specialized in non-conventional work with back patients. So, I went in for a third opinion. This MD told me he could help me get better, but it wasn't going to be easy. Armed with a list of exercises, I'd grimace as I rolled out of my bed onto the floor every morning and do my stretching exercises right there. I'd also go to massage therapy for an hour every day. The third part of my daily regimen was to walk in the pool at the nearby health club for 45 minutes per day - up and back. The water helped alleviate the pressure on my back and rebuild my strength. The club with the pool also had racquetball courts which I passed by every day during my six month rehab. I love playing and after 5 or 6 months I felt good enough to pick up the racquet again. I worked my way back into it very slowly just hitting cautiously by myself. One year after the accident, I was playing daily. Getting back on the court was a major milestone which prompted me, two years later, to write the doctor who told me I'd never play again to let him know I had just won a state racquetball title for my age group. Little did I know that returning to the court years later would almost cost me my life. That aside, beating his prognosis proved to be very gratifying. It happened because I had a step-by-step recovery plan with written goals to guide me to where I wanted to be. Do you have one of these? Part of your physical fitness plan should be to start out small and make incremental improvements every day, week or month. It can work for almost everyone. After my open heart surgery, my goal was to walk up 12 stairs by myself. Then 13, then 14, 15, etc. If the end game is to get back to a better, more active and gratifying place – on the bicycle, playing with the kids, or simply being able to take a walk or power your own wheelchair in the park – accept your own personal challenge and go after it. Even the guy at the check-in desk in the wheelchair looked physically fit. He had huge arms and could navigate that piece of equipment like nobody's business. I don't know for sure, but I bet there was a point when he had to say: "I'm going to make the best of this miserable situation."

"WAS IT OVER WHEN THE GERMAN'S BOMBED PEARL HARBOR?"

"…Hell no, and it ain't over now!" That hilariously funny and classic scene from John Belushi in the movie Animal House has been mimicked by most males under the age of 60 at some point in their lives. Sometimes car accidents and serious illnesses require a similar attitude. "…it ain't over." Looking at past triumphs can give you the confidence to know that with prayer, friends, family, a positive and determined mindset, time and physical effort, you can get to a better place and maybe where you want to be again. In my case, I understood the high likelihood that I might never play soccer or run a race again, so I latched on to the possibility of what I can do, which helps my quality of life, the quality of my health and my outlook. That said, I'm still holding onto that glimmer of hope (there's that word again) that I will be able to take a long run with my kids someday. That's hard to imagine sometimes when you can't even jog 20 steps without feeling fatigued and short of breath, but still that's always in the back of my mind as I achieve these smaller milestones. My last 5K was almost my last (as in final) race which was 4 years ago. I deteriorated to the point of zero running because my body just wouldn't do it. By the time this book was published, I could run short distances of 30 or 40 yards with enough speed to play soccer again. I have to stop after that short run and rest for a few seconds and I have to sub out every 2 or 3 minutes due to fatigue issues, but at least

I'm able to do what I love again…even though it is at a much less competitive level.

Written treatment and recovery plans not only set a course of action for healing, they also help you take an active role as an advocate for yourself in the process of getting better. Early on in my illness, after several months of test after test failing to decipher what was wrong, I put together my own treatment plan that let me measure some type of weekly improvements while also letting me test the limits of my body with very mild exercise. Although it ultimately didn't help my heart because of the misdiagnosis, it did make me feel more in control over my situation. It made me feel like I had made some progress toward getting better since it involved some minor improvements in some areas. The sad thing was that my neurologist at that time let me do it and shame on me for not taking a lesson from decades earlier when I had the car accident and found another opinion.

DO WHAT YOU GOTTA DO...
AFTER GETTING PERMISSION

OK. So the lesson learned was NOT to design my own rehab program. Now, all my exploits need to be approved by my cardiologist. Everything changed for me after I collapsed and got a top of the line, St. Jude's pacemaker. All my goals had to be reset. Getting my feet on the floor had to be Job One. Getting up and around can be difficult and maybe painful, but any physical work is also good therapy for your mind. You need activity to keep your mind sharp. A lot of the other folks on the floor spent an inordinate amount of time watching TV. I flipped on the tube only one time in my room and caught part of a show called, oddly enough, The Walking Dead. Yep, on a floor with the most critically ill patients in town, and I'm lying there watching a show about zombies. What a ridiculous waste of time. I shut the TV off and didn't turn it on again for the duration of my 9 day stay. Here's my tip on TV. If you're going to watch TV in the hospital, choose sports, something funny or something educational. Keep away from reality TV shows that bear no resemblance to reality and anything where the characters are worse off than you are.

As ordered, I got my feet on the floor and began shuffling, not walking, but shuffling my away around the floor little bits at a time. Make it to the door, then one room away, then two, then down the hall. On every stroll, pushing to go a little farther. It really comes down to being motivated to do it when you don't want to, and there were times when it got really difficult. The movement alone helps change the environment, which is why my mother and my dad ride a stationary bike for 15 minutes a day and do something called chair yoga with the other 80 and 90 year olds. (I can imagine what this looks like, just not sure I could watch it for very long.) Mom and dad both looked forward to it because it got them outside of their four walls and kept their bodies active. I'm proud of them for making the commitment to exercise every day they can. These days mom's slowed down quite a bit, but dad's daily commitment to wellness at 95 motivates me to get up and do "something" every day.

I tell my folks that they are amazing. To which they reply something like: "What's so amazing? We do what we have to do." So there it is. We do what we have to do. Most of us face some level of adversity every day. Look your situation square in the face and do what you gotta do!

WHEN'S THE NEXT WEDDING?

I said to my dad: "Dad, that's great that you exercise every day." He said he planned to keep in shape, so he could dance at my daughter's wedding. And dance he did at Daughter #1's wedding. But several months before my other daughter got married, my dad was faced with another challenge. Open heart surgery to replace a valve and a triple bypass. At age 94! (God bless Dr. Bakhos). He made it through the surgery just fine, but had a slew of other complications in the days and weeks that followed. Daughter #2 was getting married 7 months after his procedure and my dad had a similar goal. He wanted to dance at her wedding. It's important to have things to look forward to. What are the next positive milestones that you have to look forward to? Getting out of bed? Shuffling down the hall? Getting through a procedure? Seeing your son, daughter, niece, nephew or grandchild play, compete, sing, dance, get married or just telling a story? Maybe it's getting out of the hospital? If you don't have one, grab a piece of paper and calendar to write down a few. This isn't a Bucket List. It's simply a list of simple things you want to do. At the very least, it will give you something else to think and talk about.

My mom has faced plenty of medical adversity and always comes out smiling. "I like to laugh," she says. And you know what, she has a little girl giggle that always makes me smile – a positive remnant of her stroke. I talk with my mom every day and every day she gives me "advice." Good Lord, I'm well over 50 and my mom is still telling me what to do or not do, correcting my grammar, and giving me life lessons…and that makes me smile too. So, seek out things that can keep you smiling.

FITNESS: WALK IT OFF

Regular strolls around the neighborhood have now become part of my routine. After my surgeries, I would walk as much as I could because it helps my legs, heart and lungs, and it helps me tolerate my meds better. I was getting in one stroll per day, but some days I'd get in two, which left me exhausted by the end of the day. Then I'd put on the breathing mask and fight with it until I fell asleep. When the weather got cold (I live in Chicago), I'd walk in an indoor office mall that was a city block long. The morning walk was the main one. It became such a regiment that my dog, Sauté, was always poised to go as soon as I'd appear from the bedroom at the top of the stairs. (By the way, I know what you're thinking – Saute' is a really stupid name for a dog. In my defense, I didn't name her. She came with the name when we got her from the humane society. Supposedly, this is because she was a white German Shepherd and slightly brown on her back thus, "Saute." Slightly browned. Must've been owned by a chef.)

So, every morning when I came downstairs, she was frantically jumping around and giving me a look like "I've been waiting here since 3 a.m., let's go. Front door is right here. C'mon, open it, let's go." We have a route around the neighborhood that usually took us to the park where Sauté would chase a tennis ball or a stick with great enthusiasm. She was a little older, so we had to walk about a half mile before she could do her fetch routines. Yes, I had to warm up the dog for her morning exercise.

Unfortunately, she developed a tumor and fought it as best she could before she finally could not walk anymore and it was time to say goodbye. She walked by my side since the time I got sick. I miss my dog a lot and to this very day, walks around the neighborhood just aren't the same. Fortunately, I've found some suitable human replacements that have joined me on my jaunts. Most of them however, can't fetch a stick without looking ridiculous.

I still don't know what sports or activities I'll be able to get back to someday. In my mind at least, everything remains a possibility, which means there are targets to shoot for. Although, I have to be realistic. That means I might not be the same guy who could lead 8-hour training sessions on five hours of sleep – and then go for a run afterward. In those days, staying fit was what I needed to do to not be sick. I couldn't be sick because work demanded that I be in a certain city on a certain day and be "on my game" for 8 hours. I told myself I wouldn't get sick if I did certain things to stay healthy. I've since learned that anyone, no matter how healthy a lifestyle they lead, can fall ill. That's just the way it is.

In the hospital, you have a lot of time to start thinking about different things and that process continues when you are out. The questions for me revolve around where I am at physically. Am I improving? and; How do I continue to get better? My dream is to jog with my kids, play soccer with the boys from the Half Century Club, hike the Grand Canyon again (think Elise will join me if I do?), and be fit enough to do my job and chase my wife around the house. That said, it all begins with shuffling.

MARK'S RULES FOR SHUFFLING

Shuffling is something like a dance in hospital slippers while gliding on linoleum floors – a slender, attractive IV stand is your dance partner – rolling gracefully by your side. If you can get up and moving, the docs want you up and moving. It helps the immune system to work, makes you stronger, helps fight off respiratory ailments and as the nurse in my more recent stay pointed out, "can help with those bowel movements." (Why are nurse's so fixated with bowel movements?) It's not always easy, but it appears this is essential for recovery if you are capable. Yes, we're talking about shuffling, not bowel movements. Although, both are essential for recovery. Here are a few key things to know when shuffling:

Dress Code: Wear your best gown. Close it in the back to be courteous to the traffic behind you. If you have a robe, put it on. No one wants to see the crack of your dawn if they happen to be the one shuffling behind you. My attire was something worthy of a quick trip down the driveway to grab the morning newspaper – bright red checkered Mickey Mouse pajama pants and hospital gown with my very sleek beige, furry slippers. Got lots of comments on the Mickey Mouse pants, but no sponsor offers from Disney.

The Gown: Why they call this a gown, I'll never know. It's more like a smock made from a really ugly bed sheet. It has a couple of holes for your arms, and strings placed everywhere except in the place you think they should be in order to actually tie the damn thing. It comes in a variety of colors like powder blue or powder blue, and is decorated with small squiggly circles or teddy bears. It is quite the fashion statement and each hospital has it's own designer uniform for its' patients to wear, yet they all look alike. (If you go to the x-ray department, they give you a different one made out of plain construction paper...with no designs, no bunnies, and no chipmunks or lizards).

Footwear: No high heels or street shoes, please. Both are just too slippery for the floor and not the best for effortless shuffling. I had these big, stupid-looking, cream-colored suede slippers with fur on the outside. I think my wife ordered them from the Nanook of the North catalog in 1978 and now was the occasion to pull them out of storage. Match them up with my red Mickey pajama pants and powder blue gown and I was quite the spectacle. Bringing slippers from home is recommended as your feet will always be warm. Where slippers are concerned, something flamboyant and fuzzy is preferable.

Etiquette: Don't be shy. Make eye contact with the people you meet and always say hello. When passing other rooms, it's okay to give a wave to fellow patients. Ask friendly looking sorts if they'd like to join you for a shuffle. Don't forget to wear a fresh smock. You want to look presentable when shuffling past the nurses and other patients, and no one wants to invite you into a conversation when you have apple sauce and ketchup on the front of your garment.

Posture: Head up, shoulders back. My college friend, "Downtown" Al Brown has been an adjunct physical therapy advisor throughout my ordeal and always reminds me to sport good posture. Jack Chernega is a great friend and fellow skateboard enthusiast from way back in my high school days. He invented a really cool fitness product called Abdisc™ that vibrates when you slouch to remind you to sit or stand up straight. Remembering that posture is important can be hard, and I'd been slouching over my computer (or dinner plate) for so long that it was a hard habit to break. It is something I have to work on every day. Plus, you're missing part of the healing process if your head is always down and you don't see the shufflers and other folks on your route. This can also lead to IV stand crashes and personal injury…which will have the lawyers who are parked outside the Emergency Room waiting in line to talk to you about a claim. (These are the guys that usually have the billboards on the highway saying you may be eligible for damages if you've ever done something really stupid and hurt yourself, but wanted to blame someone else - even though you are perfectly fine now). Being slouched also sends a bad message to your body. You might as well wear a T-shirt that says, "I feel like crap." Posture is a physical and mental part of healing. So, stand up straight and keep your hands out of your pockets – ha, you have no pockets in your fashionable bunny-clad, drape anyway. Of course, posture is important in and out of the hospital. My wife reminds me all too often: "you're slouching." Thanks honey.

Waving: It's not quite a Queen Elizabeth wave, nor does it even have to be pageant quality. Just make it friendly; use it with people passing by your room, with fellow shufflers and any time you make eye contact with anyone on your shuffling expeditions.

Barbara was part of my frequent-shuffler program regularly joining me on my hallway tours. Being the shy one she is, and out of concern for my safety, she would keep her eyes forward or on me when we'd shuffle. Of course, I'd be looking around for someone to wave to. She couldn't believe that I would do this. "Nobody wants to talk to you," she'd say to me. Then a voice from inside one of the rooms would call out to me, "Hey, Mark, are we busting out for a beer again tonight?" which surprised the heck out of her.

Shuffling with Visitors: It was always more fun to shuffle with someone. Anytime I had a visitor, I'd say, "Let's go for a walk" and we'd go shuffling. It became therapeutic, probably for them, too, because they weren't just sitting in a chair with that dumbfounded visitor look staring at some sick guy in a hospital bed. I noticed that there were a lot of patients who were able to leave their bed and move around, but didn't want to go anywhere when they had a visitor. If someone came in to see me, my policy was to get up and go. If we didn't, we were just going to sit there, stare at each other and answer the "How are you doing?" question - which is no fun for either of us. I noticed one patient, confined to a wheelchair, was always having someone push him around the floor or to the window overlooking the garden. I told him about shuffling. And, he told me about "rolling." We exchanged tips and had a good laugh. Rolling was the extent of what he could do at that moment in time, so that's what he did. Hey, whatever works!

Get Creative: Shuffling solo or with a crew had it's difficult times, especially early on when I was testing my physical limits. You might have found me propped up against a wall or parked in a chair next to the nursing station looking like I'd just finished a marathon. There were brighter times, too. Once, toward the very end of my stay, I was feeling confident and took a soccer ball with me. My soccer friend Tony had bought it for me, saying it was the ball we'd use during my first game back. I was shuffling with it in the hall around midnight one night when I couldn't sleep. The janitor spotted me in my gown attempting to negotiate my way with my med tree in one hand and soccer ball at my slipper-clad feet. We kinda nodded to each other and I kicked it to him as best I could. He trapped it efficiently, smiled and adeptly kicked it back. We smiled, but didn't say anything. We didn't have to. It was just this neat little spontaneous exchange and made the moment fun for both of us.

"GETTING BETTER" MOMENTS

One of the key lessons I've learned going through this process is that every interaction provides the potential to feel better in some way. I call these "Getting Better" Moments. These moments happen when you look for opportunities to feel less like a sick person, and more like a regular person. There's no rule that says you can't have some fun with people while you're ill – at home or at the hospital. Well, maybe there is, but do it anyway. I'd say hello, ask if they were going to the Disney character breakfast or invite them down to the hospital pool for a swim. (of course, there was no Disney breakfast and there was no pool in the hospital). It was just a way to divert my attention from hurting (mentally or physically) to healing. And, I like to think it was therapeutic for others as well. People can be very entertaining when you give them half a chance. It doesn't take much effort to simply say hello to the people you encounter. If they return the hello, great, if not, you didn't lose anything in the process. Sure, some people are in pain or feel sick and just want to be alone. I found shuffling and interacting helped me tolerate the pain and side effects that I was dealing with much more than just laying there. Maybe it can work for you. Not everyone will give you a positive response, and some patients aren't in any position to participate, but this didn't deter me from trying again with the next encounter. And, it was fun. You never know when you can get someone to come along with you or just give them a chuckle…and many times they will surprise you and give you a chuckle right back.

So, if you are a friend or family member, offer to accompany your patient on a shuffle if possible for them to do so, or a roll if not. And, it's good both inside and outside the hospital. Outside the hospital, you'll need to set up appointments to walk with friends and family. I think you'll find it improves the experience for both of you and gives you a sense that you are taking an active role in the recovery process.

About a year after I had my open heart surgery, my father got very ill. The tables were turned now. He didn't think he could make it, but his doctors did and so did I. He spent over 40 days going in and out of the hospital due to complications and another 3 months in an extensive care facility due to requiring 24 hour nursing care. We spent a lot of time taking wheelchair rides. Just getting out of the room for a change of scenery was positive. I knew what it was like to be in the wheelchair. Eventually, he was able to shuffle a few feet. I'd encourage him to go a few feet more on each journey. We'd keep track of the distance using the 2' x 4' ceiling tiles. Now he shuffles with a walker for much longer distances. The recovery is long and there are setbacks to be sure, but progress is made and each of his Get Better Moments brings with it hope and optimism. And he is still here to see his grandchildren and great-grandchildren growing up. What a blessing for all of them…and for me.

So, be conscious of any opportunity to engage in, or even create your own Get Better Moments. I promise you'll feel better for it.

MEDICINAL MADNESS

Maybe some of you have asked: "if laughter is the best medicine, why do I need all these pills?" I was never a pill person other than the occasional Tylenol™ for a headache or Advil™ when I'd overdue it attempting an athletic movement that the wrong side of my brain thought was a good idea at the time. Funny how age and lack of agility often lose out to the laws of physics and common sense. Sure, I took vitamins and supplements to keep me healthy, which now has my friends asking, "How'd that work out for ya?" I don't remember ever taking a prescription medication before getting sick because my thought was they did more harm than good. Now, every meal looks like I emptied Michael Jackson's medicine cabinet on my plate. Like many other high-quantity pill poppers, I have two plastic pill containers labeled with the days of the week, one each for my respective morning and evening loads. Barbara has warned me about trying to restock my mini pharmacy while under the influence of my meds. This, of course, is sage advice from a woman who never gets sick or rarely ever has a bowel movement. (I'm going to hear it for revealing that last little tidbit). The meds change every so often, so it's important for me to pay attention, except that a side effect of one particular prescription keeps me from paying attention. After a visit to one of my doctors, I adjusted my dosages as ordered, except I misread my own notes and did not bother to read the label on the bottle. Instead of going from 12.5 mg to 25 mg, I ramped it all the way up to the upper limit goal dosage of 40 mg. This is great if you're into dizzy spells, blacking out or feeling like you're on the wrong end of someone swinging a Louisville Slugger™, but not if you've got a 50-something libido and are used to walking in a mostly straight line. I didn't realize my mistake until a week later when Barbara insisted on helping me fill the pill cases with the upcoming allotment. This joint discovery was immediately followed by "the look." All married men know "the look." To no avail, I tried to triangulate by pondering aloud how in the world elderly folks do this. Maybe they can see better than I, count better than I or deposit pills into small compartments better than I. Lord, I hope so, because this process takes me 10 minutes per refill and I have to double and triple check my work. I guess that's why it is important for caregivers to help with the distribution and delivery of meds. So, if you happen to see me, and I'm zig-zagging or falling over for no apparent reason, you'll know that I very likely medicated myself into the ground…literally.

MEDICINAL HOMEWORK

It seems that when you are sick, there is non-stop homework required. For me, this means sorting through the reading materials that come with my nine different daily meds. The list goes on and on ad-nauseum. (This can also be read <u>add</u> nauseum - which happens to be another side effect usually placed as a catch all at the end of the list). These pamphlets, or mini-medical encyclopedias, are the written version of those great commercials you see on TV. You know, the ones where they spend 10 seconds talking about the drug and 50 seconds speed-talking through the rest on the side effects-which always seem to include, "in some rare cases, death." Even the eye-lash growing pill could quite possibly kill you, according to the voice-over pitch woman. Although I must say that having the lovely Brooke Shields' warn you about the ultimate price you could pay for enhancing your beauty makes it somehow seem not as menacing. And a sultry voice might keep viewers listening as you hear that "some patients have experienced, nausea, kidney damage, twitching, loss of hearing, loss of continence, constipation, itchy scalp, Lymphoma and, in rare cases, sudden death syndrome." But, you will look better at your wake with those thicker, fuller eye lashes.

I'LL TAKE THE METHOTREXATE™...
AND A SIDE OF EFFECTS

There's nothing cosmetic about my med load. There's a steroid that isn't giving me a World's Strongest Man, Chinese swimmer or 1990's baseball player body. My steroid reduces inflammation inside the body, while also blowing up my face like a bright red balloon. It also made my joints sore and my stomach ache and gave me middle-age acne. The latter did at least give my 18 year-old and me one more thing in common. It's a couple years later now and I've been able to ratchet down a bit. For the last couple years, I've asked every time I see my doc if I can get off some of this stuff. I've got a Beta Blocker. I didn't even know I had Beta or why it needed to be blocked. There's also blood pressure pills to keep low what the other pills make high. I had a diuretic pill to reduce water retention and swelling that had me running to the bathroom 14 seconds after drinking anything. I take a couple other meds that one of my docs called "toxic" which is always comforting. I have to take Folic Acid to counteract something. I remember from high school chemistry that anything with Acid after it's name usually did more harm than good, but this one's supposedly harmless. Maybe they should call it Folic Stabilizer. That sounds better don't you think? Finally, there is Bayer™ aspirin because they have really good marketing. And there are others, but you get my drift. I'm a pill popper. Up to 14 pills per day depending on the day, which does lead to some interesting social interactions. 50 or 60 times a day my wife and daughters will tell me that my voice is REALLY LOUD. Or even worse, they'll tell me that they just told me something or that I was repeating myself. Blaming the meds for these last two comes in handy when you really aren't listening.

I have to take these things with food to fake my body out like: "hey stomach, here comes some mashed potatoes and no that is not Amiodarone™ coming right behind it. Just ignore that… and here's a chunk of salmon with just a dash of Lisinopril™ in the sauce that you might find interesting. That goes on throughout dinner and one can only hope that you space them out well enough so it doesn't make Mr. Stomach want to return it all to you an hour later. During dinners out with friends, I never know whether to take my drugs at the table during the salad and entrée courses, or if it's better to lock myself in a bathroom stall and take the pill regiment in private. I usually select the public dining and private dosing option.

Over time, we all learn how our meds impact us – which ones make us tired or sick or both, which ones make it hard to sleep, which ones make it hard to stay awake, which one make us pant like a thirsty dog; which ones make our nose run 24/7 like Aunt Agnes's faucet; and which one makes our tongue feel like parchment. When I first started taking them, it came in cycles. I would take the morning walk followed by my morning meds, then a few hours later, it hits and I was going down. I'd ride it out and then the upswing takes me through the rest of the day into my evening meds and bed time. Then, I got some new drugs that provided new patterns, especially on the weekends which have become a bear because of how I get loaded up on Thursday and Friday night with the once-a-week meds. When I'm transported into outer space usually sometime on Saturday night or Sunday morning, my concentration isn't the greatest. My wife explains this away with, "Don't mind him. He's on the Methotrexate™ Train."

This is another area where we all have to really work at being better in spite of what the meds are doing to us. We're competing with all these chemical reactions, which are trying to help one part of the body heal while wreaking havoc on another. The good news is that it can get better with time as the body adjusts and if the alternative is even worse, then it pays to work at figuring it out. But, you have to pay attention to your body and your bloodwork. I have to watch my thyroid, kidney, liver and onions on a regular basis. Wait, how'd the onions get in there?

We can't always control what's happening inside of us, but we can do what we can to influence the healing process. That means exercise as we are capable and when we can. It also means to follow the doc's orders, take the meds and, for me, it meant wearing the stupid mask at night for 3 ½ years. I've found that another important thing is to journal your symptoms and side effects and tell the docs. Which ones are new? Which ones seem better? Which ones are worse? This is great information. I even ask my wife what she is observing. It's all important. One more thing: Keep smiling. For those of you on the right kind of meds, this one will be really easy.

DIETARY FITNESS: HANGING OUT WITH THE PECAN SANDIE GIRL

OK, did I mention that I love to eat? Some of my meds give me a voracious appetite. Yes, put just about any type of food in front of me and I will attack it like a hyena on a carcass. One of my docs told me that I should be on a low-fat, low-salt, low processed sugar diet. OK, that's not fair for several reasons. First, I've only been on one diet in my entire life, but have stuck to it for many years. It's the Go To Bed diet. Once I stop eating for the day and go to bed, I do not eat again until I wake up. I find my intake during these periods is next to nothing. It's very effective and easy enough that anyone can do it. I magically can drop 1-2 pounds every night. Another problem for me is that just about everything I like to eat is full of fat, sugar and/or salt. My favorite vegetable is a cookie. When we'd go to the supermarket, my wife would shop and I'd go hang out with the nice lady handing out Pecan Sandies™. Barbara thought I had a thing going with the Cookie Lady. I did. I'd talk with her for 30 minutes showering her with compliments about her apron, how good she looked in a hairnet and her artistic positioning of the cookies on the tray – anything to earn multiple rewards.

If you don't care for cookies, you could try a healthier food, but it might be that something is seriously wrong with you and you need to seek counsel from a Keebler Elf immediately. It's probably nothing an entire box of Girl Scout Thin Mints or Snickerdoodles can't cure.

All that said, I do have a healthy side. It's the side of me that eats everything else. My wife works on a farm and loves gardening, so there are fresh veggies around most of the year. I like the green stuff, but am far from a vegetarian. I eat a lot of fish and an occasional steak or cheeseburger. Caring.com lists 12 "Superfoods" to strengthen your immune system. I like most of these, as well, and most can make good toppings for ice cream or pizza – and some can, in fact, be found in, or taken with cookies. The list includes: Cherries, Kiwi, Guava, Beans, Water Cress, Spinach, Onions, Carrots, Cabbage, Broccoli, Kale, and of course … Dandelion leaves. You can get the last one in my front or back lawn in large quantities. Bon Appetite!

At this point, I could probably do a whole bunch of research and give you several pages of advice on healthy eating, but I'm not going to. That would be disingenuous. One of my other docs told me that if I stay active enough, I can eat what I want as long as it is in moderation. As a rule, I stay away from high sodium or fried foods. I enjoy downing the good-for-me stuff that my loving wife serves up from her garden or brings home from the farm where she works. Or sometimes a caring neighbor cooks up a batch of something and drops some off for us. (a very nice thing for family and friends to do by the way when there is a patient in the house). So, bottom line is to go ask your doctor or a nutritionist what you should eat. Note: I find that many nutritionists forgetfully leave cookies off your dietary plan, so make sure to add them yourself if you don't see them on your list.

COACHING YOUR OWN CARING

Whether you're a caregiver, family member, friend or patient, there are times during the healing process when you have to act like a coach. I'm not talking about the guys you see on the sidelines yelling at anyone and everyone about anything and everything that doesn't go their way. We've all seen these maniacs on the sidelines who by some form of human error are granted the responsibility of "coaching" a group of little kids to learn to play "the game" properly and to the best of their ability. They rant and rave and nearly bust a blood vessel yelling at 8 year olds for not executing with perfection. These guys should be given a heavy sedative, gagged and tied to a tree 800 yards from the field of play.

When my kids were growing up, I had the joy and privilege of coaching them all – along with their neighborhood friends, to learn the game of soccer. For me, those were truly special times. Organizing a practice that would be fun, teaching fundamentals and not being so serious was my formula. Watching the kids respond was really fun. I'll bet that doctors, nurses, PT's, OT's and other caregivers feel the same way when they see their patients respond in a positive manner. Just as caregivers need to act as coaches for the patient, sometimes the patient has to act like a coach for the caregivers…to tap into their creativity, and knowledge and bring out their desire to provide patient care at the highest level.

For patients, it's a more subtle form of coaching. I'm talking about bringing out a level of patient care that is not only competent and caring, but can make you smile as well. Many doctors, nurses and other caregivers get stifled by the unwritten "rules of patient engagement." That can get them stuck in the rut of routinely just doing their job. Sure, most patients aren't going to engage their nurses, doctors and others in the same ways I did, but that's not the point. You can still be someone they want to see…someone they really care about just by being a great patient. This helps you heal as well. Patients derive great benefit from interactions outside the norm, those moments when our caregivers bring their personalities and sense of humor into each interaction…and when they give that little extra. Those get better moments are the difference makers. It's the things that patients and family members love. So, it is possible to "coach" a higher level of caring and being cared for, but someone has to take the lead. Why not you?

YOU'RE NOT JUST A ROOM NUMBER

I had a great time messing with the nurses during my hospital stays. Some would play along, while the very few that didn't just erased my playful scribbling on the treatment board and shot me a look that said: *don't you have anything better to do, like go to sleep?* Still, there were more than a few who would bring another nurse to come see the stupid things I wrote on the board or posted outside my door. If they chuckled even just a little, I knew they might be another caregiver who might see me as "Mark," rather than "8623." Now earlier, I related how conversations occur in the hallways and nurses are careful to adhere to the healthcare privacy regulations. Thus, one is required to yell "Hey Mary, 620 had a bowel movement" to another nurse down the hall instead of "Hey Mary, Mrs. McGillicutty had a bowel movement." This certainly makes sense when yelling down the hall to a co-worker is necessary. The point here is that it's much more personal when a caregiver refers to you by name. I wanted to know their names as well. Perhaps more importantly, I made sure they knew how much I appreciated their hard work and the extra care they showed me. As patients, we can't say "thank you" enough. During a routine visit after I got out, I encountered a woman in the elevator wearing a tag that read ICU Nursing Manager. She looked like she needed to fall asleep for a week. I decided to tell her how great her nurses were, naming individual women and how they were the best. This woman just started beaming like a proud mother. With nurses like: Sarah, Megan, Lucie, Kelly, Amy, Lisa and Dara, she should. Lucie was the first nurse I met when I arrived and to this day when I see her at the hospital, she always asks how I'm doing. Sarah proved herself to be a spectacular trainee, a ray of sunshine. Every time she came in the room we had a great conversation and lots of smiles. If that goes with her into the next room, and it becomes OK for her to do that as part of her approach, then she's now better at her job. I simply hope an overzealous supervisor doesn't squelch her enthusiasm. Megan and Dara were seasoned pros, the perfect balance of pleasant with a high degree of professionalism and competence. They took the time to explain things to me on my level rather than in medicalish or medicinalese, two languages invented apparently for no other reason than to overcomplicate something that is already complicated and to keep the average person from understanding what was going on...and they put up with my antics. I see Megan once a month during my volunteer days at the hospital and we've become friends. She is a truly wonderful person, as are most of the nurses I was fortunate to be in the care of at Edward Hospital. They helped me through a difficult time by being better at their jobs than someone just going through the motions. If you gals are reading this, I love you all and thank you from the bottom of my enlarged, granuloma-filled heart.

Oh, remember the story I told you earlier about my hair washing day? Later that same night there's a knock on my door. "Come in," I said, expecting it to be someone wanting to stab me with a needle or make me take another pill. "I understand you had a special order for Fresh Grapes," the food service worker said while presenting me with two bowls of grapes. (This is what I'd written on the treatment board under 'Sponge Bath and Massage.) No matter how I felt just before she walked in, at that very moment, I couldn't help but smile. I felt better. I had just been on the receiving end of another Get Better Moment. I guess I'm not just a room number after all.

IF THERE'S ANYTHING I CAN DO...

If you've been paying attention, you already know the first question everyone is going to ask you: "How are you doing?" Now, let's talk about its counterpart, the parting comment you'll usually get toward the finale of a visit or conversation: *"If there's anything I do to help, just let me know."* It might sound like a formality, but most people really are coming from a genuine place when they say this. My standard, jovial, response usually involved inviting the questioner to clean my gutters, mow the lawn, black tar my driveway or take my hospital gowns to the cleaners. Hey, they asked, right? But there is an even better response.

The truth is that you know the comment is coming and you know the person asking it, so have an answer that not only can help you with healing, but that also fits who the caregiver is. Again, we're looking at the type of friend they are – faith, business, sports, fun – and asking something of them they can realistically deliver. This goes for family members as well. If you know they are devout, ask them to pray with you and for you. If you know that they believe in God, but don't go to church very often, ask them to attend a service on Sunday and pray for you. (That helps you both). If it's a business acquaintance, ask them to help you with something business related. For friends living elsewhere, send them a note and maybe add something funny. Ask them to return the favor. If you're in the hospital or homebound, you have plenty of time to think and plan how friends, neighbors, co-workers and family can help you.

How you use that time is either going to help you heal or not. Watching TV and trying to guess the next letter on Wheel of Fortune is a mind-numbing waste of your time and won't help you much…unless you plan to go on Wheel of Fortune.

For me, the health of my business became something I thought about while incapacitated. I'm not the first business owner to have health issues, but I wonder how many turn to their friends and co-workers for help during this process? You might have to. Many folks get into the sick mode and it becomes easy not to think about other things. It's extremely important to think about other stuff because it distracts you from discomfort and negative thoughts, all of which helps you fight through your illness. So, I focused on ways to keep business moving without me out there beating the bushes. I met a business friend shortly after getting out of the hospital. My response to his "What can I do" question was ready. I asked him to reach out to his business contacts with a short email (that I had written up in advance) that explained what my company does and for them to give us a call if we could be of assistance. It would be helpful, really helpful, to sign on more customers, and this happened to be an available route for doing that while I was out of the picture. Now, you have to be OK with asking for help because it might not be the easiest thing to do. But, if the business friend truly wants to help, and I believe they do, I've just done something that's pretty painless. And, I made it easy for them by writing up the note for them to send. It's up to them at that point. Then, I hand it over to my staff to get it done and keep us up and running and send a thank-you note expressing my appreciation for their help.

Some folks really deliver without even needing to be asked. My business friend of about 20 years, Terrence lived in Wisconsin and drove to Chicago to see me after I got out of the hospital. He told me he would do one of my presentations or even create a presentation for one of my audiences at no charge.

That was his gift to me while I was not working. Wow, that was impressive. Even more so because Terrence is really talented. He would have enjoyed doing it and I know this offer came straight from his heart. And, he even brought some delicious pastries when he came to see me. Bonus!

Not everyone has a business, but the main message remains the same while in or out of the hospital, and that is to let your friends know what you need to get better. Maybe watch your dog or cat, or look after your plants. Help you write some cards or emails. Collect your mail. Mow your lawn. Whatever.

For me, helping my business along would reduce stress, and anything your friends can do to reduce stress helps the healing. Got a friend who makes you laugh until you cry? Ask them to send you a funny story – or a humorous book, perhaps. My college crew – George, Paul, Murph, Jim, Eddy J, Joey Z and Dave – consistently send me funny emails stories and jokes. Most live far away, so I don't get to see them very often. When they asked what they could do, I told them to keep me laughing, and they have. And I tried to encourage their silliness by sending them humorous replies that poked fun at my own situation and the events going on around me. Some of the stories in this book (like the Sleep Clinic and Dermatologist) were sent to the guys as I was writing them. There isn't a week that goes by without receiving something ludicrous from someone in the group. And by returning the favor, you keep the string alive. I love these guys. They help me more than they'll ever know.

This one is important. Tell your friends that you don't mind if they let others know what's happening and how to get in touch with you. Let the magic of the Internet work for you. One fraternity brother I hadn't seen or heard from in many years sent me a stupid, silly email card because I told my core group it was OK to let others guys in on my situation. Three guys that had been notified by "the crew" stopped by to check up on me when they were in Chicago for business. Chalk up 3 more getting better moments.

Spelling out what you need in your recovery is equally, if not more, important once your road to healing takes you out of the hospital. Something changes with your family and friends when you're at home healing. They want you to get better. You want to get better. So, help educate them on what your recovery entails and the role they can play in that process. And, funny as it sounds, if you are in the hospital, telling visitors when it's time to go is something else you can't be afraid to do. Some family and friends will stay past our point of exhaustion, and you or your hospital room wing man just has to gracefully dismiss them. Do it nicely and invite them back. Thank them for coming and let them know how you need your rest and how it'll be no fun for them to be sitting around when you fall asleep mid-sentence and start drooling.

GETTING OUT AND ABOUT

Remember when hanging out with your friends meant more than anything else in the world? In high school, maybe you'd go grab a burger, head to a sporting event, or go to the mall or movies. In college and your 20s, it was probably hanging out in someone's apartment, or a bar or restaurant. Everyone loves being part of the group. That doesn't change just because you're in your 50's and having heart palpitations that can jump start a Mazda.

For my mom, it was her bridge group, for some the Garden Club, Book Club, Health Club or Bible study group. For me, it's my soccer team. During my first season on the sidelines (not playing – just on the sidelines), I couldn't drive. One of my teammates picked me up and took me to the game so I could watch. It was the first time in months that I had been back out there, albeit in a chair under an umbrella on the sidelines. I had a great time seeing the guys, talking about the game and just feeling like they were glad to have me there. Being out there was part of the healing process for me. They kept asking how badly I wanted to play. Man, I really wish I could have been out there. I'd hate for that ball they gave me in the hospital to sit unused for too long. A while later, one of guys from soccer called and asked if I wanted to join them at a sports bar to watch one of the European Premier League matches. Sure, they knew I couldn't help them finish off a pitcher or two, but it was great to be invited despite being sick. And, watching your friends cuss at the TV can add some humor to your day. It turned out to be a great time and we've done it a couple times since. I was away from the game for almost 4 years during my recovery, but able to maintain a connection. For me and my recovery process, it was important.

If you're a friend, don't assume the patient doesn't want to get out and about because they're going through an illness. It helps if they tell you, "Hey, give me a call and let's go out," but approaching the topic can be such a morale booster for the person trying to heal. They might turn you down or sound like they're making an excuse not to do it. Be prepared for that, and try to find ways to draw your recovering friend out of their bubble. If the patient is in a wheelchair, offer to push them around for a change of scenery. If they can't get out of bed, ask them what movies, shows or pictures they might like to see.

Once the recovery process shifts to the home front, it gets more common for the patient to let the bubble surround them. For me, the easy route would be to get up in the morning, take my meds and go back to bed. In fact, I could go take a nap right now, but I know I have to move. You just don't want to be languishing around the house all day because that can get depressing fast. Maybe some folks need that comfort or need the opportunity to sleep. I understand that, but also understand the need to get out, get some fresh air and interact with folks. Feeling like you've accomplished something by the end of each day is also a healer. Ask, how can I feel better today? For me, that meant spending some time at the office — if I could catch a ride with someone. Now I can drive again, so that's a lot easier. I'll schedule a breakfast or lunch with a friend. I invite people to join me on walks. I'd get out to every one of my kids' sporting events before they went off to college. Soon, I'll be volunteering more at the hospital. Whatever it is I can do that pulls me out of the house, sign me up, let's do it. There is one I wasn't so sure about. My wife signed the family up to go dog sledding in Minnesota after Christmas. I guess freezing to death in some godforsaken wilderness, hundreds of miles from civilization while tied to the front of a sled makes for a better story than: "He went to sleep one night and never woke up." Thankfully, my doctors nixed that idea, so the kids went on the 3-day jaunt in minus 6 degree weather and my wife and I hung out at the cabin, walked around the town a little and watched some movies. That was an intelligent alternative to frostbite and death by mushing.

When you think about it, getting out and about has its place in the hospital as well. I didn't want to sit in bed watching TV or just lie around waiting for the next shots, tests or meals, which is why shuffling around became so important. First, it got my body moving. Second, my travels created a chance to interact with other patients. Maybe one of my floor mates would see me shuffling by and yell out "Hey Mark!" I'd stop in and they'd turn the TV off for a few minutes so we could talk. Don, the church usher was unable to walk. However, he'd ask me in to chat when he saw me shuffling by. Once he asked me to talk with his grandson on the phone to describe his upcoming angioplasty. There was a trust established that allowed us to communicate and gave him the confidence to ask me to have that phone conversation. Another time, we talked for a while about all the jobs he had living in our town. None of this would have happened if I didn't get out and about, or if Don didn't respond to my outreach. We established a bond through a common experience that was far greater than the passing head-nod hello's we'd share at church.

Now that I am somewhat functional again, it's easy for me to say, "get up, get out and get going," but I understand that not everyone can do it so easily (or at all), and I've been there. For some, you might only be able to move from the hospital bed to a wheelchair. Great, if you can get to the chair, ask someone to take you somewhere else, even if for only a few minutes. And, move your mind even if your body can't. If you drift or become unmotivated, it makes it so much more difficult to get better. Use the 5 F's to find the ways you can improve with every day – even if it's asking others to help you make it happen.

When my dad got sick and was confined to bed or a wheelchair, my sisters and I would wheel him out to the pond near his convalescent center and enjoy some fresh air. A few times, I'd bring a fishing pole and toss it in the water. It broke up the monotony of recuperating in a stark stuffy room.

FEELING CONNECTED

When things get tough it's always great to have a friend by your side. I never expected my closest friend to be going through his own serious medical issues at almost the exact same time my heart troubles peaked. I introduced Dave earlier. He and I met as fraternity brothers and have been best friends ever since. It's weird to use his real name because we've stuck to nicknames for so long. He's definitely in the league of great guys for so many reasons, especially his outrageous sense of humor – something we both appreciate. The doctors feared Dave had a brain tumor, although thankfully it turned out to be an abscess. However, it still required a serious course of treatment, including brain surgery to remove the abscess and multiple IV drip treatments every day for three or four months. That's brutal and onerous. He used that sense of humor of his as a mental fitness exercise to keep his head right for dealing with it. One time, he wrote me about going to a play that his daughter was in and how he took pride in knowing there'd be lots of other guys there wearing ball caps, but he'd be the only person in the audience with a metal plate in his head. He just flat out makes me laugh; we tell jokes and stupid stories every time we talk on the phone. Sometimes, I've got tears in my eyes by the time we're done making fun of our situations and each other. At the end of the day, Dave and I know we've helped each other in our own unique way. Those moments add up over time. We know how to be serious, too. I asked him, "You're a strong guy mentally, how are you coping with all those drip treatments?" Without a flinch, he said it's what he had to do as part of the new routine. This chapter in our friendship was a bit different because neither one of us could do all the things we wanted to do, yet that all gets put in the background when we talked on the phone. Thankfully, he's since healed and is back to normal. Still, having a connection with someone who knows firsthand what it is like to be unsure of your future can be comforting. It's good to know that you're not in the boat alone.

It's pretty easy to look around and see the friends you have great connections with. Again, it's about knowing how each person can help you get better on your road to recovery. Along that path, there are many other connections and friendships which will appear, even if for only a short time. I was really disappointed when fellow ICU-er Bob left the hospital. He was two doors down from me, so it was fun for me to shuffle down there and just cut up with him for a few minutes each day. One time we were laughing so hard, I guess his monitor went off and the nurses came running into to make sure Bob was OK. "Yeah, we're OK. Just going over the daily activities," he said. We were talking about the Lunch n' Learn on How to Work the Damn Bed when we lost it big time. As a patient, I also got to be a friend to others who were in the same boat as I. We all held the common thread of having serious problems. Bob and I built a kinship out of this, just as Don and I did. Don was quite a bit older than I am, so the stakes of his trip to surgery were high. He didn't know how things would turn out and was scared. As a friend, you have the ability to provide a high level of comfort to people, to help them prepare for the best possible outcome or, in some cases, whatever the outcome might be.

TRY ONE OF THESE

There's also a camaraderie that connects patients, families and caregivers. We're all in different cabins on the same cruise and can band together in support of one another. Making my shuffling rounds one time, I saw a bit of a commotion down the hall. I was told to return to my room because they had to do emergency surgery right then and there on the floor to a man who was 4 or 5 rooms away from mine. He wasn't going to make it to the OR. He was hooked up to every manner of medical device. He survived the emergency surgery. Bottom line is that he was beating the odds. He was incapacitated in his room, but surrounded by family members who all sat silently looking very grim. A day later, I stopped by to see how he was doing and we talked about how strong he was, that he was putting up a great fight. A few simple words from some stranger they'd seen slowly pass by their room many times seemed to bring some comfort to his wife and relatives. We talked for a while and the conversation brought a smile to the wife's face. It might have been one of the few smiles she had that day. Everyone in that room was very serious because the situation was very serious. His wife and relatives offered a kind smile every time they saw me after that point. One day they invited me into the family waiting room where they were all having lunch. We shared some stories and they wanted me to try some of the traditional foods that they brought. Meeting his family was important to me. Those brief interactions were definitely "getting better moments" because they had me thinking about someone other than myself. It was interesting how a connection grew out of a couple brief moments spent together. When you make the attempt to reach out to someone in need, sometimes they reach back. Maybe they even take your hand and in that moment, perhaps it helps in some small way. If so, that's a good thing. Another lesson learned. I think every time we do something to help another person get better, we get a little better ourselves.

The other obvious connections, if not momentary friendships, you can make are with the caregivers. I'm convinced that being friendly with the nurses and other hospital workers helps you feel better. I'd ask them about their families, their birthdays, and things like that to get to know who was taking care of me. Try to go out of your way to be nice to all your caregivers, and not just because they are sticking you with needles and pumping you with drugs, but because they have tough jobs and are trying to do their best to help you or your loved ones. Introduce your caregivers to the important people in your life, whether that's your family or any person who comes in to visit. It's a vital thing to do because of how it builds a stronger connection to you as a patient. In my case, my docs and nurses saw they weren't just working for me, they were working for my wife and four kids as well. You can hear and feel the difference in some of the conversations once those introductions and connections are made. If nothing else, get to know your nurses because you are going to see them more than just about anyone else during your time in the hospital. Even today, when I run into the nurses that took care of me, they always ask about my family. As you can see, "friend" has a loose definition in the world of Getting Better. It can be anyone who has the ability to help you not only feel better, but maybe even be better.

MEET SARCASM, ZOEYGIRL2, M2000, AND FARINA

When I was first diagnosed with Cardiac Sarcoidosis, I didn't know what to do. I'd never heard of this disease or known anyone who had it. The online articles I read painted a very bleak picture. I was worried for my wife and four kids, and for myself as well. One of the places that I found to get help and meet some new friends was on an on-line support group. The one I use for my disease is Inspire.com. You can search for almost any illness and find people who are struggling and looking for answers just as you are. Spouses and family members can join in as well. I've learned a lot from the people on this site and made some long distance friends in the online support group that I've never met face-to-face. Some want to vent. Some need support. Some are looking for answers. Some want to share their story and know that they are not alone. Some share their experience or knowledge about the disease and treatments. Others provide encouragement. Some are funny. Some are serious. Some are healing and some are suffering. All are related by disease. I've come to like these people even though some are only known to me by their user ID. Others become more open as we both share our experiences. The courage and compassion of my fellow patients in this community truly do inspire, as it is so aptly named.

On this site you will find all 5 F's present and accounted for.

- People of Faith share the strength they get from their belief in God.

- Families draw knowledge, strength and support for coping with their sick loved one.

- Patients become Friends and bring each other comfort.

- Tips for physical and mental Fitness help keep the mind and body strong.

- There are even patients sharing jokes and funny stories for those who want to have a little Fun.

There is an annual conference that focuses on this rare disease that this online community has. It encourages patients, families and friends to attend the event, with speakers who are doctors renowned for their special knowledge of the disease and its treatments. I attended one and had an opportunity to meet some of the faces behind the names. Not real names, but everyone uses online monikers like: AuntBev, StopThisNow, CardSarc, GreenParrot, Chemical and JoyBunny. I wish I could meet them all. I feel like I already know some of them. Maybe another part of getting better is sharing experiences with people who are going through what you are going through. People who know the pain and frustration of dealing with, and recovering from the same thing you are. Meeting this many fellow patients for the first time also adds some fun and anticipation to the healing process. I smiled a lot, shared some funny stories, asked a lot of questions and hugged some folks who have been through a lot of heartache – literally and figuratively. If you're at the next one, look for me. I'll be the one in the bright purple shirt that reads: "We're Getting Better!"

PATIENT'S BEST FRIEND

I attended Fr. Pat's church one Sunday. In his homily, he was making a point and jokingly asked the men in the congregation: "If you locked your wife and your dog in the trunk of your car for 10 hours; when you opened the trunk, which one would still be happy to see you?" Of course, we all laughed and thought...how true. Maybe you have a pet that you can play with, talk to and care for, just as they are caring for you. During my illness, one of the constants was my dog.

I introduced you to Saute earlier. Like many family pets, she was thrust upon me by my kids who promised to feed, walk and care for her. Well, like most parents that are dumb enough to believe this ploy, guess who ended up getting up with the dog at 3 or 4am to let her out, walking her every day and playing fetch with her? Yep, yours truly. So, by default I became very attached to "my kid's dog."

As long as you treat them well, dogs will love you unconditionally. Any time you come home is cause for tremendous celebration. When I came home from the hospital, the dog went crazy, tail wagging, whining, jumping all over. You get the idea. To my dog, something wonderful had happened and it was for her, the most exciting of moments. Master had come home. Of course, the same thing would happen when I returned from a 5 minute outing to grab some ice cream at the local grocery store. To dogs, every happy moment is the best and happiest moment of their life. Maybe there's a lesson there for all of us regardless of whether you're sick or healthy. Trying to make the most of every waking moment is a pretty good habit to get into.

According to WebMD, pets can help humans to: reduce stress, lower blood pressure, increase social activity, be happier, be less lonely, and even live longer. Certainly, my Saute helped with all this and she played a key role in my recovery. Now that I think about it, I'm not sure if I walked her or she walked me. She couldn't wait for me to come downstairs in the morning because of the thrill associated with the first event of the day – our morning walk. If I tried to sleep in, there she would be, nose to nose with me at my bed checking to see if I was OK and thinking… *"Hey, get up. It's time for our walk. You can throw some sticks in the school yard and I will fetch them. This is going to be so much fun."* 3 or 4 sloppy face licks later, I was coerced out of bed and out the door.

I mentioned earlier that my companion developed a tumor and her health failed quickly. It was hard to see her sick and unable to do the things she loved to do. Maybe my family went through the same thing watching my health fail. It wasn't long before we had to take her to the vet for the last time. I tried to be macho dad, but must admit, losing my dog brought me to tears.

Failing health takes everyone involved on an emotional roller coaster. In the last few years, I've experienced most of the emotions - good and bad, that go along with recovery from illness. My companion isn't here to take me on walks anymore and I miss her presence. She helped me through a very difficult time in a number of ways. She even had a sense of humor, pooping every day on the same neighbor's lawn who kept a particular political sign in their lawn supporting a politician of dubious competence and integrity. It always made me laugh and yes, I removed it…not the sign, the poop.

Whether you have a dog, cat, bird, or whatever, I'm sure you get some recuperative benefits from the little creature. Do you think they know how much we appreciate them? Maybe so, and perhaps it reminds us to tell our family and friends who help with our healing just how much we appreciate them. And, we can take them along on our walks as well…but, they usually won't fetch sticks.

MY RANDOM ACTS OF STUPIDITY TOUR

I'm no daredevil, and I didn't even realize that I was putting my life on the line every day during the first 10 months of my illness doing the unthinkable – walking up stairs and attempting to play recreational sports. Like many of us that get hit out of the blue, I had a time bomb in my chest ready to go off at any moment and I never knew it. Ignorance + Denial + Bullheadedness = Stupid. And as Forrest Gump used to say, "stupid is, as stupid does." As doctors tried to figure out why my body would inexplicably shut down and recharge, I did like any good performer would and kept going on with my act. After all, the show must go on right? Wrong.

The first of my almost-final performances was for a limited audience of one (Elise) on a huge stage, the Grand Canyon. Eight hours of hiking while fighting for breath and experiencing pure exhaustion made for high drama. And, when I emerged, it wasn't long before I felt like nothing had happened. Why go to a doctor? I had to have another near-death experience while running a 5K race with my boys. One might call this another stop on Mark's Random Acts of Stupidity Tour. It took that incident to get me in for a checkup. But, the tour continued.

There were dozens of negative test results and months of misdiagnosis. During this time, the docs had me pumped up with a daily dose of steroids to fight what they thought I had. It masked some of my symptoms and made me feel artificially and temporarily better, though far from better. I got impatient and the soccer field was the next stop on the tour. I couldn't play my usual game anymore because it exhausted me just trying to run a short distance. Unwilling to acknowledge the problem enough to actually stop playing, I did the second-most logical thing: I switched to defense, so I didn't have to cover as much territory. Run 20 to 30 yards (as far as I could go), stop, pass the ball, and catch my breath. On the inside, something was tick, tick, ticking away, but I kept going. It wasn't long before I couldn't run at all and had to quit.

Doctors spent months trying to figure out why my body drained of energy faster than batteries in a kids' toy on Christmas morning. They swung and missed a few times before thinking they figured it out. Wanting to get back on the stage again, I concocted my own treatment plan to get me doing all the things that made me feel like me. I thought that if I tried to jog a little faster…or a little farther, it would help me outrun my problem. Ok, so this proved to be another really bad idea. But, no one told me that. In fact, one neurologist told me to "go ahead and see how it feels." Advice that could have killed me. My heart was on overload.

What very nearly turned out to be the final act for a cat that had used up 8 of his 9 lives came on that racquetball court in tournament competition. Sure, I had been hooked up to a heart monitor for the previous 24 hours, but I wasn't going to wait for test results or ask permission from doctors who might say, "No, you can't do that." Against all basic common sense and wisdom, I played. That was my award-winning, knucklehead move. If only I could have realized that before all of my breath left my body and I collapsed.

The problem all along was hiding in my heart, which seemingly revved itself to levels not seen on most EKGs or Indy 500 race cars, for that matter. In the early stages, not knowing what really was wrong meant my doctors and I were treating something I didn't have. It turned I was doing myself much more harm than good. Denying the reality that I wasn't getting better certainly didn't help either. My intentional push-the-envelope attitude made me the poster boy for the "Don't try this at home" (or outside the home) campaign.

If you're listening to your body and it's telling you something is wrong, then investigate it a lot further, rather than letting it go or testing it to the point of collapsing. Just as I switched to defense in soccer to compensate for my struggling health, people have a tendency to treat illness with a defensive approach. That includes trying to sort out your problems yourself or ignoring them in the hope they'll go away.

Now, if you've got a definitive diagnosis and a physician-approved plan for an at-home therapy to get better, go with it and work hard. If you're just trying to work through something on your own, you're basically just mixing chemicals and swallowing it down, hoping tomorrow will be better. Home therapies truly only work to the extent you're treating the right thing. Odds are against your personal treatment plan being successful. If you don't know what you have, you're shooting in the dark. And, when you shoot in the dark, you can wind up getting to go for a ride in an ambulance. I learned this lesson the hard way.

In spite of my best efforts to accidentally terminate my existence, I'm still here to tell you my tale. Don't join me on tour and don't follow my early examples – except for the going to the doctor part, that is.

MY CREDO

In so many ways, this book has been cathartic for me. In the early days of my illness, it helped me categorize and understand what I needed to do to cope with the realities of my situation and the unwelcomed events that invited and continue to invite themselves into my life each day. So many of these ideas have enhanced my relationships with people that I care a lot about. And they've allowed me to share a smile and a kind word with people that I'll cross paths with perhaps only once. My hope is that in some way the ideas, stories, strategies and 5F's will give patients, family members and friends something to think about. At times, I've contemplated what happens if I don't get better. Those are the times when I need to remind myself that even if I don't heal – I can still get better in other areas. I can grow in my Faith. I can commit to stronger relationships with Family and Friends. I can still find ways to enjoy the day. And I can look for laughter in the face of it all because that is what I've decided to do.

I'll give you my rationale for <u>living</u> as best I can.

My heart is damaged and my body is weak, but my outlook is healthy and my resolve is strong. I will get better.

I can no longer do many things that I want to do at the level I used to do them, but I will do the things I can with joy and enthusiasm. I will not be denied happiness.

I'm not the same as I was, but I am still here. I hope that in some ways, I am better.
My eyesight is diminished from age and the drugs I take, but I will continue to look for ways to be stronger in my Faith, and become a better husband, father, and friend.

Sometimes news is negative, but I hope to have a positive influence on the people I meet in the hospital, at work, at play and in my community.

I will not take what I <u>can</u> do for granted, as there are always others far worse off than myself and my wish is that they can get better, in some way, as well.

I will strive to live each day to the best of my abilities, and if someday I can no longer maintain the fight, I'll know that I've gone down swinging with a smile on my face and no regrets.

I will pray to God daily with thanks for the gift that is each new day. Amen.

WHAT'S NEXT?

As patients, we're always looking to answer the question: "What's next?"

I started to write this book 4 years ago. During the early months of writing this book, after my discharge from the hospital, my progress had been phenomenal. I was beating my doctor's expectations and thinking that I'd be back to normal in a year or less. Then, several months later – much to my disappointment – I started to rapidly decline. They implanted a pacemaker/defibrillator device in my chest to save my life and it still keeps me going today. After a time, I learned that the disease had ravaged the right side of my heart which was dangerously enlarged due to exertion and I also had severe tricuspid valve damage. The doctors said that they needed to go in and perform open heart surgery and perform a rather tricky procedure to repair this valve. Left untreated this all would lead me to a place that is not on my vacation list. Two words that I feared were "heart transplant." If my open heart repair procedure didn't work, my cardiologist told me that this might be in my future. Former Vice President Dick Cheney waited 20 months for his transplant, but I didn't have that kind of time. My hikes in the Canyon tell me that you have to get to the top before nightfall. Despite a few complications, Dr. Mahmoud Bakhos at Loyola Medical Center was able to pull it off. He opened my chest and spent several hours putting Humpty Dumpty back together again. The man is a genius and I have to place him high on the list of doctors that I owe a debt of thanks to. So, my climb out of this predicament now becomes a hike that includes maintaining an aggressive med plan, regular testing and evaluations, doing everything possible to keep the disease from spreading to other organs, constantly working on my mental fitness to remain positive and doing what I can to be physically prepared for whatever comes my way next.

One of my mantras has always been "Pray for the best, but prepare for the worst." I pray a lot more these days – for my family, my friends who are ill and for myself. I've made the decision to go forward with a smile, to focus on the 5 F's and get better in every area possible. I try not to dwell on the things over which I have no control. I don't see any gain in looking back and I don't know what the future will bring, so the focus is on each new day. It sounds trite, but each day truly is a blessing, so my objective is to do something worthy of being here and thank God for the privilege of waking up to do it.

Like all of us, I don't expect the worst, but I've talked to the insurance agent, the lawyer, the financial planner and the accountant to make sure my wife isn't burdened by extra hassles should the worst come to be. It eases my mind to know those details have been addressed. My financial advisor tells me of a client's father that had no will and did no estate planning which left their affairs in quite a mess and created havoc inside the family after his passing. Don't let that be you. It's actually quite comforting to know that everything is in order.

From now on, I will let my guard down and tell my family and friends about the path ahead – good and bad. And, they'll also know I'm still going to live my life to the best of my ability. I never thought I'd be in this position, but here I am. If you are a patient, you might have thought the same thing. In that case, we are together. You are not alone.

It is a comforting thing to know that we don't have to fight sickness alone. We can enlist the aid of: family and friends, caregivers and new acquaintances – even those we never actually meet, and most importantly, God is always there for us especially when we are left to our own thoughts or when we think we are in this alone.

We can find help in person, over the phone and even on-line. I'm so thankful for the people in my life that pray for me, walk with me, send me notes, call me out of the blue, tell me jokes, work to heal me, and are themselves patients, perhaps like you, who are inspirational examples of how to live a meaningful life despite their condition. It's also important to remember that living a meaningful life can also mean that your life is meaningful to someone else – someone who draws strength and inspiration from you. You see, this book is about your story too. You have different experiences to share and stories to tell. Do your children or grandchildren know your story? Have you shared the lessons learned and values that have governed your life? Do the people you care about most know how much they mean to you?

I pray that most of you are on the road to recovery while understanding someone reading this may be looking at nightfall coming sooner than expected. Just remember: Yogi Berra famously said, "It's not over 'til it's over." This book was designed for all of us – healing or healthy – to look at the 5 F's: Faith, Family, Friends, Fitness and Fun and decide how to use some or all of those pieces to make ourselves, a loved one, or a friend get better.

I hope *Getting Better* brought a smile to your face and gave you a few helpful things to think about as you navigate your way through your own healing process.

So, keep the faith, hug your kids, kiss your special someone, call a friend, pet your pet, eat healthy, research your condition, get out of the bed, play your favorite song, walk if you can, be strong, think positive, grab a cookie, have some fun… and keep smiling.

Let's all Get Better.

EPILOGUE

I started writing this book in Feb, 2012. My circumstances kept changing requiring multiple rewrites and in January, 2015, my dad became very ill giving me a different perspective looking at healing from the caregiver point of view. I've tried to be sensitive to what family and friends see and can do when someone they care about is injured or ill. Getting better is a day-to-day process. Over 4 years after my breakdown in the Grand Canyon, I stepped on the soccer field again. It was exhilarating. I can't run as fast and can only go for a very short time before the heart and body tells me it's time to catch my breath and recover. Nonetheless, I am out there playing again with a great group of guys all over 50 who are trying to recapture their glory days. Most of my medical advisors thought the possibility of this to be remote. Remember to ask the question: Is it possible that I will be able to...?

I now feel like I am getting better. Of course, there are still hills to climb and I still have "those days," but overall I am functional and my doctors have not recently had to take any body parts out of me or put any foreign metallic items into me. The results of my most recent tests have been encouraging instead of discouraging. And speaking of hills to climb, I started an annual fundraising campaign where I will be climbing 100,000 stairs in landmark locations across the US to raise awareness and funds for sarcoidosis research and patient assistance. That was impossible to think about just a short time ago when I couldn't walk up more than 7 stairs without my body failing. I am only one of thousands who have had remarkable recoveries and beaten the odds. Maybe you can too.

I'd like to hear if you used any of the prescriptions in this book or any other self-prescribed solutions to get better. Please make a comment on my website at: GettingBetterWithMark.com.

Let's get better together.
God Bless,
Mark

THANK-YOU'S TO MY MEDICAL TEAM

Dr. Costanzo: Thank-you for having me as your patient, for guiding my care and for caring. I can't imagine where I'd be if it wasn't for you.

Dr. Bakhos (and your team): Thank-you for your skill and attention and for giving me a new lease on life. Everyone kept telling me you were the best. There's no doubt in my mind. And thanks for saving my dad's life as well.

Dr. Greenstein: Thanks for equipping my chest with that pacemaker/defibrillator. I've been putting it to good use.

Dr. Sweiss: Thanks for your ongoing efforts to look for clues to conquering this miserable disease and for your guidance, concern and prayers for me as your patient.

Dr. Pappas: Thanks for your watchful eye and being that trusted second opinion early on in my illness and as you follow my progress. I'm glad to have you in my corner.

Dr. Nemivant: Thanks for the phone calls and the extra mile… even when you were on vacation. And most of all, thanks for giving me permission to put the CPAP machine in the closet. (My wife thanks you for that one as well).

Dr. Franklin: Thanks for the fact that you always make time for me, and for your willingness to help me every which way.

Dr. Baughman: Thanks for your research efforts. May you find the breakthrough.

Dr. Ahmad: Thanks for putting my eye back together in time for my daughter's wedding. You are truly an artist.

Lucie, Megan, Dara, Amy, Denise, Sarah, Big Mike and the rest of the Heart Hospital nursing and care staff at Edward Hospital. Thank-you for your amazing care and for putting up with my antics. I love you all.

Tish, Rose, Brian, Nikki, Handmaa and the rest of my care team at Loyola Medical Center: Thank-you for getting me up and going. You guys were awesome.

Brett and Shelley: Thanks for the timely and flawless execution of all my prescriptions and your smiles every time I come in.

GETTING BETTER GETS EVEN BETTER

Follow our progress and let us know about yours!
Please check out our website at GettingBetterWithMark.com to see updates and follow Mark's progress as he works his way around the country on his Climb For A Cure. We encourage you to leave a comment on the website if you wish and to follow Mark on Twitter and Instagram: @mlandiak

Getting Better Keynote and Workshop Presentations
Mark now spends some of his time presenting his unique prescription for wellness as a Keynote and workshop speaker at meetings and conferences for companies, hospitals and associations. To talk with Mark about a presentation at your upcoming event, send Mark a note on GettingBetterWithMark. com, call 630-778-9991 or email: mnigro@CorpDyn.com

Additional Book Orders
You can use the GettingBetterWithMark.com website for orders of 24 or less, but for bulk orders of 25 or more, call 630-778-9991 or email: mnigro@CorpDyn.com

Donations
We encourage everyone to consider a contribution to the Foundation for Sarcoidosis Research by going to StopSarcoidosis. org and clicking on "Join The Fight," then "Donate Now." FSR is a registered 501(c)3 non-profit organization. Your contribution is tax deductible to the full extent allowed by law.

Printed in the United States
By Bookmasters